The Evolution of a Medical Center

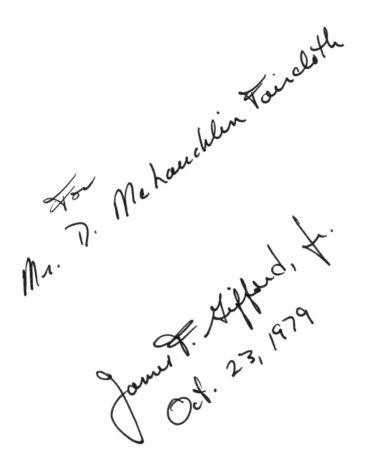

For
Mr. D. McLauchlin Faircloth

James F. Gifford, Jr.
Oct. 23, 1979

The Evolution of a Medical Center

A History of Medicine at Duke University to 1941

James F. Gifford, Jr.

Duke University Press   Durham, North Carolina   1972

© 1972, Duke University Press
L.C.C. card no. 73–185464
I.S.B.N. 0–8223–0290–x

Printed in the United States of America
by Kingsport Press, Inc.

To Clarice

Preface

The complex of health care institutions provided for the Carolinas by the philanthropy of James Buchanan Duke had its origins in a set of four factors. Chronologically, these were the medical poverty of the rural South, the standards of medical education set by The Johns Hopkins University School of Medicine, the desire of James B. Duke to arrange his philanthropy so that the profits derived from the natural water resources of the Carolinas would be directed to the social needs of their residents, and the economic circumstances of the great depression. Within these limits the Duke University School of Medicine and Hospital, in cooperation with The Duke Endowment, transformed the practice of medicine in the Carolinas from a decentralized cottage industry into a modern integrated network of health care facilities and in the process shifted the financial responsibility for adequate medical care from local practitioners operating private hospitals to the general public. This process of modernization, largely accomplished within the professional lifetime of the originating faculty of the School of Medicine, made the Carolinas' experience a forerunner of national medical development and conferred upon the Duke University School of Medicine and Hospital the status of a national medical center.

This book is the first of two projected volumes intended not only for residents of the Carolinas interested in their local history but also for medical educators and social scientists concerned with the changing forms of medical education and the delivery of health care in the United States. It traces the social origins of the rise of Durham, North Carolina as a regional health center and describes in detail the philosophy, funding, administration, educational theories, research objectives and regional aid programs of the Duke health care institutions up to the outbreak of World War II. The dislocations caused at Duke by that war and the major changes in national medical objectives, supporting agencies and educational patterns which followed it make 1941 the most logical date to end the first volume. Although by that time the Duke health care facilities had earned a considerable national reputation, the focus of this book is regional throughout.

This study took three years to complete, and involved more persons that I could ever thank. Professor I. B. Holley, Jr., gave me countless hours of assistance from the inception of this work to its conclusion: to him are due thanks not readily expressed in print. Professors Richard L. Watson, Harold T. Parker and Robert Durden, Drs. Barnes Woodhall, David T. Smith, Wiley T. Forbus and E. Croft Long, and Mr. Elon Clark, all of Duke University, read parts of the manuscript, offered constructive criticism and became valued friends. Mr. G. S. T. Cavanagh, Miss Mattie Russell and Miss Kathryn Kruse provided major assistance in locating and compiling the material on which this study is based. Mr. George Watts Hill opened his family archives and with them new perspectives on the history of Durham. Messrs. Marshall I. Pickens, James Felts, George Harris and the late Dr. Watson S. Rankin guided me through the voluminous records of The Duke Endowment. Finally, many members and former members of the faculty of the Duke University School of Medicine contributed their recollections to this story. Among these were Drs. Jay Arena, Joseph W. Beard, Frederick Bernheim, Mary L. C. Bernheim, J. Lamar Callaway, F. Bayard Carter, George S. Eadie, Julian Deryl Hart, Duncan C. Heatherington, Angus McBryde, Elbert L. Persons, Robert J. Reeves, Robert A. Ross, Julian M. Ruffin and Warner L. Wells. None of these persons, of course, is in any way responsible for any errors of omission or commission which may remain in this work. To all of these, and many others, I am grateful.

My thanks go also to the Josiah Macy Jr. Foundation for a grant which supported the major portion of my research and writing, to Duke University for financial assistance during the first stages of the work and to Dr. William G. Anlyan, Vice President for Health Affairs of Duke University, who was instrumental in securing funds in support of publication. Without the help of these and many other individuals this study long ago would have been abandoned.

My thanks go finally to my wife, Clarice Mason Gifford, for the untiring assistance in research, editing and typing, as well as for unswerving support.

James F. Gifford, Jr.

Guilford College
1971

Contents

Illustrations

Part One: Origins, 1865–1931

Chapter 1: The Agricultural-Industrial Frontier: Durham, 1865–1889

When Hiram V. Paul wrote the first history of Durham, North Carolina, in 1884 in praise of the industry and virtue of her leading citizens, he could boast of every phase of her development except her health conditions. The two decades following the Civil War saw Durham grow, on the popularity of bright-leaf tobacco, from an insignificant railroad hamlet of less than 200 inhabitants to a manufacturing center of over 5000. Six major factories competed for larger shares of the market with innovations in advertising, mechanization, and price reduction, then absorbed smaller competitors as Durham's industrial revolution entered the consolidation stage. As the factories prospered and population increased, shops and services of all sorts multiplied, a lyceum was established with the ultimate purpose of establishing a public library, and the town's leading Methodist industrialists sponsored a female seminary. Only the reputation of being one of the most unhealthy spots in the state marred Durham's success story.[1]

Although bright-leaf tobacco was increasingly popular in the South before and during the Civil War, the importance of Durham as a center of the industry nationally was the product of historical accident. In the closing weeks of the conflict Generals William T. Sherman and Joseph E. Johnston, the commanders of Union and Confederate armies in North Carolina, met west of the town in a small farmhouse owned by James Bennett and there discussed, prematurely as it turned out, terms for an end to all hostilities.[2] While the commanders conferred Durham and the surrounding area were declared neutral ground. Troops of both sides rifled the supplies of John R. Green's, Durham's only tobacco factory, and the barns of surrounding farms, carrying away large quantities of bright-leaf smoking tobacco. When these troops were mustered out scant weeks later, they carried Durham tobacco throughout the country. Soon orders for more, addressed to the postmaster, railroad agent, and other town officials, began to pour in. Green seized his opportunity, branded his product "Durham Smoking Tobacco," established a bull as his trademark, and resumed manufacturing.[3]

Green's business grew rapidly, not only because his brand of Durham tobacco was first in the market but also because his trademark, the Durham bull, immediately caught and held the attention of the individual customer. In 1868 he took in as a partner William T. Blackwell, tobacco jobber from Kinston, North Carolina, who in turn purchased the entire business for $2850 when Green died in 1869. In its first year the W. T. Blackwell firm, owned by Blackwell and James R. Day, produced 33,000 pounds of "Bull Durham Smoking Tobacco." In 1871 Julian S. Carr, an advertising expert, joined the firm, purchasing a one-third interest for $4000. Through personal salesmanship, lavish entertainments, premium gifts, endorsements by prominent personalities, and widespread advertising featuring the bull in a variety of poses in various types of periodicals, Carr exploited the chance popularity which the war had given Durham tobacco.[4] As "the Bull's" sales soared, other firms began to sell "Durham" tobacco and to use a bull on the package. In a lengthy series of court cases, however, Blackwell's won the right to exclusive use of the bull and the word "Durham" was restricted to brands manufactured in the Durham area.[5] Blackwell's began to dominate the market. In 1878 a one-third interest in Blackwell's sold for $94,000. By 1882, when Carr bought out Blackwell, the same interest was worth $150,000.[6]

Blackwell's closest Durham tobacco competitor was the family firm, W. Duke Sons & Company. Washington Duke, the head of the family, was a Durham farmer who foresaw the importance of bright-leaf tobacco and converted his assets into tobacco holdings prior to his enlistment in the Confederate army. Released from a Union prison at the end of the war with fifty cents in his pocket, he returned home to find that most of his hoard had been appropriated by the armies of Sherman and Johnston. With his three sons, Brodie L., Benjamin Newton, and James Buchanan Duke, and a daughter, Mary Elizabeth, he processed and packed the remainder in a shack on his farm and labeled the product "Pro Bono Publico." The profits saw his family through the winter and encouraged him to continue to manufacture tobacco while at the same time working the farm to provide food for his family.

In a small log cabin on the farm he and his sons produced about 15,000 pounds of smoking tobacco in 1866, shredding and packing the leaf in their "factory" whenever the weather did not permit working the farm. In a full day they were able to manufacture 400 to 500 pounds of smoking tobacco. The finished product sold for fifty to sixty cents a pound, of which about twenty cents had to be paid out in revenue taxes. By 1872 the family farm factory was turning out about 125,000 pounds of smoking tobacco per year. In 1873 Washington Duke purchased land in Durham at a cost of $500 per acre and erected a factory at a cost of $1500. On one side he and his younger sons made "Pro Bono Publico" and on the other his eldest son Brodie, operating independently, manufactured "Duke of Durham" smoking tobacco.[7]

The Duke firm benefitted from court decisions which allowed any Durham resident to use the words "Durham smoking tobacco" on his products,[8] but the most important reason for the success of the company in its early years was James B. Duke's personal salesmanship. Soon after moving to Durham, Washington Duke had taken James Buchanan and Ben into the firm as partners. On the road beginning in 1875, James B. or "Buck" visited wholesale and retail customers alike "as long as the stores were open," thereby reducing the company's reliance on commission merchants and wholesalers.[9] In person and in print he tried to counter the idea that Blackwell's alone produced genuine Durham tobacco. His sales forced the firm to seek new capital to buy raw material. In 1878 W. Duke Sons & Co. was formed with capital of $70,000. Brodie Duke's firm, producing "Duke of Durham" tobacco, was absorbed into the family business and George W. Watts, son of a Baltimore tobacco merchant, was added as an equal partner. Two years later Washington Duke temporarily retired, selling his interest to Richard H. Wright, another Durham tobacco manufacturer. With James Duke operating the factory, Ben Duke handling business correspondence, Watts acting as treasurer and Wright traveling and selling, the firm expanded. In 1879 Watts hoped to double their trade over the preceding year, and by 1881 the firm had far outstripped all other Durham concerns except Blackwell's.[10] James B. Duke, however, was not content to stand second to anyone. "My company is up against a stone wall," he remarked. "Something has got to be done and that quick. As for me, I am going into the cigarette business."[11]

Cigarettes were a gamble in 1881. Scarcely more than 400,000 had been made in the preceding year, mostly in New York, and their hold on the American public was tenuous. Four Durham firms, including Blackwell's, began to produce them at the beginning of the 1880's, but only James B. Duke staked his future on them.[12]

Duke hired European cigarette rollers away from the New York concerns which had recruited them abroad to come to Durham to supervise his new operation and to train local workers in the art. A skillful roller produced 2500 to 3000 cigarettes a day. When Congress voted to reduce the revenue tax on tobacco from $1.75 to $.50 a pound in 1884 the Duke firm cut the price of its cigarettes in half even before the tax reduction took effect, making their packs the cheapest on the market and radically increasing demand.[13] Advertising tactics were roughhouse. Edward Featherston Small, the Dukes' star salesman, opened the Atlanta market to the firm by obtaining the endorsement of a popular French actress, placing a painting of the actress with a package of W. Duke Sons & Company cigarettes at one of Atlanta's busiest intersections under the caption "Atlanta's Finest," and then purchasing all available billboard space in the city for thirty days so that other firms could not counter. James B. Duke personally scrutinized every detail of the promotion, demanding from his drummers not only orders from retailers but also reports on how many customers were calling on the retailers for Duke cigarettes and how sales of Duke cigarettes by each retailer compared to sales of competing brands.[14] In April, 1884, the company told Small:

> Our cigarette business was never so good, orders ranging from 200 M to 400 M daily while the Bull has purchased stamps this month for only 250 M altogether, if you mention this do so in confidence or you might get our Collector in trouble. We are getting up circulars for each retailer you sold in Atlanta with their names and addresses on & hope to get them ready next week & are also preparing some other physic for the Bull which we will administer from time to time.[15]

To meet the demand the Dukes built a new factory and on April 30 James B. Duke installed the first Bonsack cigarette machine to be used in North Carolina. Invented by a 22-year-old Virginian, James

Bonsack, this machine was then capable of producing 120,000 cigarettes in ten hours, the equivalent of 48 hand-rollers, provided it did not break down.[16] Duke spent many hours working with Bonsack and a young mechanic named William T. O'Brien in improving the performance of the machine. The cost of rolling cigarettes fell from 70 cents a thousand to 25 cents, and the profit per pack to the manufacturer, according to Small, approached 100 percent. Even before the machines were perfected, however, their necessity was obvious. The firm was doing business at the rate of $200,000 annually.[17] Orders poured in from every section of the country where the drummers introduced the cigarettes. Even with the Bonsack machine and the entire factory working at capacity the firm was almost 7,000,000 cigarettes behind its orders by October, and feared that "friends may become disgusted and decline in future to handle Duke cigarettes."[18]

James B. Duke himself, however, had already left North Carolina for New York City. With $75,000 in risk capital he proposed to open a factory to compete with established New York firms for the northern cigarette trade and to relieve the Durham factory of 300,-000 to 400,000 cigarettes a day.[19] His concentration upon cigarette manufacture using intensive advertising, demand analysis, elimination of middlemen, machine production, and price reduction proportionate to tax relief had brought the tobacco industry to the brink of revolution.

Duke's departure ended the first phase of Durham's industrial development. She now was growing faster than any town in the state. As a consequence the problems of water supply, sanitation, and overcrowding common among towns on the frontier of the industrial revolution became more and more serious. Living conditions were— and were felt to be—actively offensive and inconvenient. Water from private wells, rising amidst garbage dumps and privy middens, often was impure. In the absence of water works and a sewerage system, mild cases of typhoid fever were so common as to be called "Durham fever." Epidemics of malaria, dysentery, and diarrhea visited the town periodically. The "immense volume" of tobacco dust raised by the factories was considered a health hazard, and among factory workers at least, the incidence of tuberculosis was reported high. The Board of Commissioners took little corrective action: not until September, 1883 was it made illegal to allow hogs "to run at large in the City." Champions of other towns made much of these conditions as compared to their own.[20] Although one Durham health officer pleaded with the Commissioners to publish the town's mortuary statistics, "thereby preventing slander against the health of our town," there is indication that Durham's favorable position compared to other towns was the result of incomplete records.[21] There were no hospital facilities.

Durham's Board of Commissioners faced the agonizing question of what to do first. Outside developers were eager to provide the town with an adequate water supply. Some of Durham's leading citizens, led by Dr. Albert G. Carr, brother of the president of Blackwell's and personal physician to the Duke family, pressed for construction of a hospital. The local newspaper, *The Durham Tobacco Plant*, had as its motto "For Durham agin the world" and, as that might imply, championed both causes. The water supply, justified not only as a matter of health and cleanliness but also in terms of fire protection, convenience, and civic pride, received first priority. The choice proved politically astute when a series of destructive fires and a number of deaths from typhoid fever occurred during construction. And as *The Daily Tobacco Plant* pointed out, nearby Winston, North Carolina *already* had a water works. The town fathers would not go so far, however, as to approve the municipal sewer system which the water works made even more necessary,[22] and bowel diseases remained prominent among the causes of deaths in Durham.[23] The committee appointed to investigate the hospital project never officially reported back to the Board.

When his search for financial support through the political authorities proved fruitless, Dr. Carr attempted, beginning in February, 1888, to raise the necessary funds through the Durham Medical Society. The Society appointed a committee "to invite the cooperation of the different churches, benevolent orders, prominent citizens, and the county and town commissioners in a movement looking to the organization of a Hospital Association and the establishment of a hospital for the benefit of the poor."[24] Hospital drives commonly suffered from the idea that hospitals were places for the indigent; persons of any substance were cared for at home. The Durham "poor," however, included the young factory workers with neither home nor relatives in the community who were "often left to care for themselves upon sick beds in back rooms over stores, in private boarding houses, etc."[25] Durham numbered more productive poor in her population than any other city in the state, and for this reason the plea for hospital facilities received an initial hearing on moral grounds.

The plan was warmly applauded but poorly subscribed, perhaps in part because no epidemics came that summer, with only a few cases of malaria and diphtheria reported. The largest contribution, other than an initial donation of $100 by the Durham Medical Society, was $50 by the Knights of Pythias.[26] *The Daily Tobacco Plant,* fearing that Durham would fail to keep "fully abreast with our neighboring communities in all that constitutes a first-class town," offered to pay the first year's rent on any building suitable for hospital purposes "provided satisfactory arrangements for the maintenance and support of the hospital can be entered into on the part of the town, the ladies, and the physicians."[27] When no agreement was reached on a suitable site, Dr. Albert G. Carr offered the Society either of two lots owned by him, one of 2.38 acres and the other of five acres, providing that a hospital building costing $3000 be placed on the first or one worth $10,000 on the second.[28]

Durham's men of means, however, preferred to invest their extra capital in an exposition intended to attract statewide attention to local industries and stores, and thereby to avoid the effects of the general business depression then gripping North Carolina. The exposition paid for itself and drew up to 15,000 visitors, but soon thereafter 17 businesses failed, including W. T. Blackwell's bank, which had overextended credit. Durham's commerce was not seriously hampered, but for the first time since the Civil War her citizens lost their confidence in the future, and with it went all chance of raising large funds through private donations.[29]

W. Duke Sons & Company was not touched by the wave of failures. Willing and able to cut prices to meet all competition, the firm grew rapidly after James B. Duke moved from Durham to New York. In 1885 the firm was incorporated with a paid-in capital of $250,000.[30] James Bonsack repaid James B. Duke for his help in perfecting his rolling machines by guaranteeing Duke a rental 25 percent below that charged any other manufacturer. When the European rollers in Durham threatened to strike against or destroy the Bonsack machines, they were replaced with local labor. James B. Duke himself invented a pasteboard box with sliding cover to replace flimsy paper packages for cigarettes, and when the public accepted this innovation, machines for stamping and packing the boxes were added to Duke's production lines.[31] In his first year in New York, Duke's machine-made produce won a large share of the market from the supposedly superior hand-rolled cigarettes of other Southern firms. Although the company produced 2 million cigarettes daily by July, 1887, it was 10 to 12 million behind orders and buying raw materials so heavily it was barely able to redeem its notes and keep a bank balance.[32] By 1889 W. Duke Sons & Company produced at the rate of 940 million cigarettes annually, or nearly half of the nation's total output. The firm paid $600,000 in taxes and spent an equal amount on advertising. With such sums at his command James B. Duke already was making plans to eliminate the need for such expensive advertising by bringing his four leading rivals into a combination under his control.[33]

The lesson of these events was not lost on Dr. A. G. Carr. The town, the ladies, and the physicians could not raise the money necessary to give Durham adequate hospital facilities. Only the tobacco magnates, Julian S. Carr of Blackwell's or the partners in W. Duke Sons & Company, might provide sufficient funds. Brother of the first, friend and physician of the others, Carr turned his attention to pleading Durham's health care cause in private.

Chapter 2: The American Medical Revolution: Medicine at Trinity? 1889–1923

In the civic competition among North Carolina cities at the end of the nineteenth century Durham suffered the reputation of a parvenu. To overcome this, provide for the needs of a growing population, and give expression to philanthropic impulses and religious convictions, Durham's tobacco magnates provided the city with both a college and hospital facilities. North Carolina physicians, prominent among them Dr. Albert G. Carr, attempted to unite the state's chronic need for physicians with the social service tradition of Trinity College, primary philanthrophy of the Duke family. Five times in three decades the hope for a medical school in Durham surfaced. Each time, however, the cost was more than Trinity could bear because, in those same three decades, American medical education underwent a major revolution.

Durham residents got the first hint of the events which would change the character of their community on May 25, 1889, when *The Daily Tobacco Plant* published a plea by a Trinity College alumnus to other alumni to rally and prevent the removal of the College from the small Randolph County community of Trinity, North Carolina.[1] Durham Methodists knew the College well. From its beginnings as a subscription school supported by Methodist and Quaker farmers willing to educate their children, it had grown into a normal college, or teacher training institution, which also gave instruction to Methodist ministers free to gain the financial support of a Methodist constituency. Finally it had evolved into a Methodist liberal arts college which trained businessmen and lawyers as well as preachers and teachers. Since most rural North Carolina Methodists were poor, three trustees, among them Durham tobacconist Julian S. Carr, were supporting and managing the school in 1887 when John Franklin Crowell became president.[2]

Fresh from Yale, Crowell sought immediately to increase the constituency of the school and balance its budget by building on and publicizing Trinity's tradition of training men for public careers in law, medicine, politics, business and religion and thereby, in time, attract public notice to the College. To fill the gap until his students were established, Crowell himself publicized the College by writing pamphlets and delivering lectures on the need for economic and social progress throughout the state. One address, recommending state levies for schools, highways, railways, river control, seaport construction, and a survey of the state's economic resources, was reprinted as an open letter to the General Assembly of North Carolina at the suggestion of former Democratic Congressman Furnifold M. Simmons.[3] He also frequented professional meetings, gaining attention for the college by soliciting suggestions on how Trinity might better prepare her graduates for their careers. His contact with the medical profession led to the introduction of special preparatory courses in pharmacy and medicine in the Trinity curriculum. Although neither of these programs survived more than one year, Crowell became known in the state as a man with new ideas who was interested, as he put it, in "improving the general health of the population by means of scientific health instruction as a branch of the social and economic sciences."[4]

Crowell was convinced that "to place Trinity in the front rank of American Colleges" he must move it to a central city, where an "aggressive" college could raise more funds, hire better qualified faculty and secure more able students who in turn could enjoy a wider social experience and gain practical training in the public professions.[5] After educating Trinity's trustees concerning the consequences of urbanization he placed Trinity on the market as a prize in the civic competition among North Carolina cities. An opening bid of $20,-500 and a site, which would have allowed Trinity to duplicate her facilities, was received from Raleigh, North Carolina's capital, in June of 1889.[6]

Almost immediately rumors of a counter-offer from the city of Durham were heard. Raleigh had recently acquired the Baptist Female Seminary (now Meredith College) despite Durham's offer of twice as much money because Raleigh seemed a more suitable city for ladies. The civic pride of Durham's leaders suffered a severe blow. Also, North Carolina's Methodists were divided into eastern and western conferences. A move to Raleigh would take Trinity out of the western and into the eastern conference. Washington Duke, staunch Methodist and loyal Durhamite, was persuaded by his son Ben, who was a trustee of Trinity College, and Methodist ministers

R. F. Bumpass and E. A. Yates, that it would be best for Methodism, for the people of Durham, and for the College if Trinity moved instead to Durham. After meeting with Crowell in January, 1890, he offered to guarantee $85,000 for the buildings and endowment and Julian S. Carr donated the fair grounds west of the city as a site for the school.[7] Crowell readily accepted, feeling that "old things had passed away, and, behold, all things were becoming new."[8]

For Dr. Albert G. Carr this news brought new possibilities. In addition to his concern that Durham have hospital facilities, he shared with other North Carolina doctors the fear that North Carolina's chronic shortage of physicians might become critical. Prior to the Civil War the state's doctors trained largely as apprentices in the homes of established practitioners. The few whose families had sufficient means studied in the medical schools of the North, or in Europe, and returned to play prominent roles in the affairs of the State Medical Society. After the Civil War, however, it became clear that graduates of apprentice relationships possessed uneven skills and that schools outside the region would not supply North Carolina with adequate numbers of physicians. The state's first medical school, in what is now Hoke County, founded in 1866 under the name Edenborough Medical College, expanded the residence concept by allowing as many as eight students at a time to observe the practice of its founder, Dr. Hector McLean, who operated the school to increase his income. Graduates were only as well trained, however, as the limits of McLean's practice allowed. When the school failed to survive his death in 1877, members of the medical profession began to petition the General Assembly for state regulation of medical practice and to seek a lasting solution to the problem of physician supply.[9]

The second attempt to solve the problem began in 1879 when Dr. Thomas W. Harris was persuaded to move his private medical school from Chatham County and graft it onto the permanent structure of the University of North Carolina at Chapel Hill. Harris was appointed to the faculty, without salary, and taught, virtually by himself, a two-year preclinical medical curriculum including courses in anatomy, chemistry, botany, physiology, materia medica, therapeutics, and the practice of medicine and surgery. At the same time he operated a weekly free clinic where students could see, and under his supervision treat, minor illnesses.[10] The school lasted six years, finally failing because Harris neglected his classes to make a living from his practice, lacked wide support among the state's doctors, received little help from the University, and failed to get his students admitted with advanced standing to northern medical schools.[11]

The University trustees quickly moved to replace Harris's proprietary school with a genuine University medical course because of the demand from local doctors and from students studying outside the state, some of whom testified that Harris's course gained them at least a year's start on other medical students. Dr. Richard Whitehouse was called from the medical faculty of the University of Virginia. Under his direction the University's preclinical course gradually attained high standards, its graduates being readily admitted to the third year of northern medical schools without examination by the turn of the century.[12]

By now, however, a number of North Carolinians had awakened to their need for increased medical services. The Honorable A. H. A. Williams, Mayor of Oxford, North Carolina, welcomed the thirty-seventh annual meeting of the State Medical Society to his town with these words:

> Why is it that in a profession thus amply supplied as is the Medical Faculty of North Carolina . . . there are so often various types of patients who must of necessity seek medical treatment beyond the limits of the State . . . ?

> The objection that much money is taken from the State, never to return, is secondary in comparison with the inconvenience, annoyance, and other disadvantages that are transparent on a moment's reflection. Among these disadvantages the sparseness of population, the lack of large cities, and the dearth of money are hinderances not readily surmounted, still I opine that much at no distant day will be accomplished through your honorable organization to overcome these difficulties.[13]

It was in response to this sort of interest, expressed widely across the state, that a group of North Carolina physicians, including Dr. A. G. Carr, frustrated by the failure of the State Medical Society to sanction more than a preparatory medical course at the University, began to look for an independent location for a full-fledged medical school. In March of 1891 they met with Crowell to discuss the possibility of establishing such an institution in connection with Trinity College.[14]

Crowell recognized immediately the desperate need for more physicians for the state. In 1890 North Carolina stood sixteenth among the states with a population of 1,617,949. To serve these people the state had 1294 physicians, a ratio of 1 to 1250, placing North Carolina forty-first among the forty-five states for which such figures were available. In addition, the percentage of these doctors who lacked formal education was so large that standards for licensure passed by the General Assembly could not be enforced. Even when such practitioners were prosecuted under existing laws, grand juries refused to indict them because in rural areas ill-trained doctors were regarded as better than no doctors at all.[15]*

The physicians proposed to Crowell a medical school with professorships in Anatomy, Physiology, Practice, Surgery, Materia Medica, Obstetrics, and Chemistry, to be housed in separate buildings for which, they hoped, "such a man as Dr. John Franklin Crowell" could raise funds. A "first-class" hospital would be built in connection with the department. The General Assembly, they suggested, might so arrange it that a graduate of the program be granted license on his diploma, thus encouraging local students to attend the school and, by so doing, saving North Carolina the export of an estimated $50,000 yearly in medical education costs.[16]

The medical needs of the state and Crowell's dream of an expanded Trinity were perfectly compatible. On April 7, 1891, Crowell produced a "Plan for the Inauguration of a Hospital and Medical College in Trinity College at Durham, N.C. beginning with the fall

* The laws of North Carolina as of 1858 established a Board of Medical Examiners composed of "regularly graduated physicians" to examine and authorize doctors to practice in the state. The only penalty for not having a license from this Board, however, was not being able to sue or recover before any court on a delinquent medical bill. Practice without the license was finally made a misdemeanor in 1889, and a fine of not less than twenty-five nor more than one hundred dollars or imprisonment could be levied. J. M. Baker, ed., *The Constitution of the Medical Society* . . . , pp. 3, 6. Not until after the turn of the century, however, did licensing laws begin to drive quacks from the profession in North Carolina. See James A. Burroughs, *Needed Legislation and a Practical Enforcement of Existing Laws*, pp. 13–14, 18–19.

term, October 1, 1891." He envisioned a new classroom building, to be provided at a cost of $3000 by the Trinity trustees, and the conversion of two existing residences. The trustees also were to guarantee an annual income of $2000 to the resident surgeon and resident physician who were to have charge of the hospital. For these funds Trinity was to draw on the income of the hospital, fees from students for medical care, and voluntary contributions. Any fees from private practice were to be figured as part of the salary. The two physicians were to manage the hospital and teach the first two years of the medical curriculum, assisted by two members of the College faculty, one in Biology and Physiology, the other in Chemistry. After two years three additional chairs would be added, in Practice and Pathology, Surgery and Gynecology, and Diseases of Children and Obstetrics.[17]

Crowell's plan foundered both because it failed to win the backing of the State Medical Society and because the depression of 1891–92 choked off funds from Trinity's Methodist constituency. The proposal that a diploma from the school should guarantee a state license to practice medicine drew heavy fire from Medical Society president Richard H. Lewis and other members who were fighting for tighter licensing laws under the supervision of the medical profession itself. They also opposed supporting another school unless the salaries of the staff and departmental expenses were guaranteed from endowment income and thus not dependent on student fees. Finally, they held that no city in North Carolina had a sufficient population to provide an adequate base for clinical study. When building costs at the new Durham campus exceeded estimates, the project was doomed. As the college opened in its new Durham campus, in September, 1892, the Trinity trustees were again struggling to keep the doors open.[18]

During the same period in which James B. Duke's family secured Trinity College for Durham, he himself moved to take control of the entire American cigarette industry by bringing together the five principal domestic cigarette manufacturers, including W. Duke Sons & Co., in a new corporation, The American Tobacco Company. With authorized capital of 25 million dollars and exclusive rights to the Bonsack rolling machine, the new corporation produced 90 percent of all cigarettes in the United States. Duke then moved gradually to acquire control of important manufacturers of plug tobacco, cigars, smoking tobacco and snuff. Once he achieved control of the manufacture of all major tobacco products, he moved into production of raw materials and retail marketing. By 1906 American Tobacco had no serious competition; its securities had a total value of $255,000,000 and the company was still expanding.[19]

Although James B. Duke until 1903 devoted his full attention to the expansion of the American Tobacco Company, Durham's resident tobacco magnates began to turn profits from that industry into allied enterprises. The Dukes, Watts, and Julian Carr contributed large sums to and were active in the formation of companies which built new railroads for Durham. Ben Duke, Brodie Duke and Carr each capitalized a cotton factory in the town. These at first manufactured bags for the tobacco factories, but gradually grew and produced a wide range of cotton goods. Ben Duke's investment in Erwin Mills of Durham and his holdings in mills in other cities eventually made him one of the largest promoters of the cotton manufacturing business in North Carolina.[20] Around tobacco and textiles, other related industries developed. Watts's brother-in-law, Lewis A. Carr, led in the development of the Durham Fertilizer Company. Between 1890 and 1900 the assessed valuation of property in Durham more than doubled, and the population rose 45 percent. Wealth remained, however, in the hands of a few. Not until after the turn of the century did minor industries which catered to the local needs of an industrial community flourish and small enterprises in general gain a substantial basis.[21]

Increasing wealth brought increasing irritations to the Dukes who remained in Durham. During the agricultural depression of the early 1890's small farmers suspected the large manufacturers of profiting excessively at the expense of farmers. Warehouse operators, who were the immediate object of the farmers' wrath, worked to direct that hostility toward the American Tobacco Company "trust." In addition, appeals for charity poured in from indigent folk throughout the state, each one asking for a loan or a gift. Some were worthy, but many were not.[22] The tax structures of the state and county were not as advantageous to the Dukes, with their large holdings of stock and securities, as were those in some other states. In a letter to a business associate B. N. Duke wrote:

Confidentially, I do not see how we can live in North Carolina. I wish you would, at your earliest convenience, find out about the local taxing laws of New Jersey, and whether or not private stockholders of the American Tobacco Company would have to pay tax on their certificates . . . I am getting tired of blackmailers and robbers in this town and county, and I do not see how we can longer submit to it.[23]

The Dukes were similarly dissatisfied with their connection with Trinity College. In the spring of 1890 B. N. Duke had threatened that his family might "wash our hands of the whole affair" when a Reidsville newspaper publisher, who had attacked the Dukes both as operators of the "trust" and as Republicans, was given a place of honor at Trinity's commencement. The failure of Methodists to contribute to Trinity's endowment led Washington Duke to feel in 1892 that his gifts were not appreciated, and the failure of Trinity to meet its budget for faculty salaries made B. N. Duke, who managed the family's local philanthropy, feel that funds were being mismanaged. Late in May, 1892, he resigned as a member of the Board of Trustees.[24]

Ben Duke grew increasingly sensitive, however, to the financial problems of Trinity's rural Methodist constituency brought on by the agricultural depression. When Crowell demonstrated his good faith by hiring an agent to collect debts owed the college and made an effort to fund its floating debt, Ben Duke rejoined the Board of Trustees and, with the help of George Watts, engineered a sale of college bonds which maintained Trinity during the depression years 1892 to 1894. His decision to remain in Durham was no doubt helped along by a Durham County tax ruling which assigned no value at all for tax purposes to his family's common stock certificates and assessed preferred stock at the rate of valuation of 20 cents per dollar of face value. In 1894 John Carlisle Kilgo, a Methodist preacher noted for his fiery oratory, replaced Crowell as president of the college and reunited Washington Duke's religious zeal with the desire to place Trinity on a firm financial footing. By 1900 the Duke family had contributed almost half a million dollars to the college, and their giving inspired other donations. As the century turned, Trinity was financially secure.[25]

The uneven distribution of wealth had for many years made it all but impossible for local hospital fund drives to succeed.[26] In 1895, however, the personal efforts of Dr. A. G. Carr, who was unsuccessful in earlier attempts to have a hospital erected by the city fathers (1884), by popular subscription (1888) and by Trinity College (1891), finally were rewarded. Out of gratitude to the people of Durham for their friendship as well as a sense of Christian steward-ship George W. Watts, president or director of tobacco companies, cotton mills, railroads, and a bank, decided to make a large philan-thropic gesture of benefit to the townspeople. The excellent nursing care he had received during an illness in 1892 initially directed his attention to the desirability of building a hospital. Tours of Durham and Dr. Carr's entreaties convinced him of its necessity.[27]

Watts presented Durham with a completed five building "cottage hospital" on February 21, 1895. The complex included an admin-istration building, male and female wards, a surgical suite, and autopsy and mortuary facilities. Equipment for the hospital was patterned after that used at The Johns Hopkins Hospital in Balti-more. Eighteen of the twenty-two beds were "free"; that is, open to any white person in need of care absolutely without charge if neces-sary. Watts Hospital was the first private hospital in North Carolina offering completely free care to those unable to pay. The cost of the buildings and equipment was approximately $30,000. The remainder of his $50,000 donation Watts placed as an endowment on the hospital, expecting that this would yield $1200 toward an annual budget of $4000. Control of the hospital was vested in a board of trustees, four to be appointed by the Watts family and one each by the Methodists, Missionary Baptists, Presbyterians, Protestant Epis-copalians, the town, the county of Durham, Trinity College, the Academy of Medicine, and the Watts Hospital Association, a group of citizens who raised funds for the hospital. By giving each of Dur-ham's major institutions a share in the control of the hospital Watts hoped to insure that neither "party-politics, sect, nor clique" could gain control of the "people's" hospital.[28] The first trustee he named, himself excepted, was his partner, B. N. Duke, who immediately used his influence to insure passage of the hospital charter by the General Assembly.[29]

The people of Durham initially harbored mixed feelings about hospital care. The city government voted $1200 annually toward the budget and private donations of cash and furnishings flooded in, but in the first nine months only 68 patients came for treatment, and Watts was disappointed by the lack of patronage. Hospital care still carried connotations of charity and, more important, of impending death. There were, however, only three deaths at the hospital in those first nine months, and satisfied patients gradually added their public encouragement to that of the town's physicians. Watts Hospital became the first general hospital in North Carolina to be rated "Class A" by the American Medical Association. The reappearance of typhoid in the town resulting from lack of adequate sewerage facilities also increased the number of patients. By 1901, when the health and welfare of Durham were "jeopardized by the prevalence of Small Pox within and near the corporate limits of the city," most citizens had no hesitation about hospitalization.[30]

The renewed outbreaks of contagious diseases made Durham's citizens pay attention to the need for hospital facilities for Negroes as well as whites. Since 1893 the city's leading Negro physician, Dr. Aaron Moore, with the support of Dr. Carr, had been soliciting funds. Once again, however, it was essential to secure large donations from wealthy, which is to say white, citizens. In the past Washington Duke had expressed a desire to erect on the Trinity campus a monument to the memory of Southern Negroes who had remained loyal to Southern whites during the Civil War. Drs. Moore and Carr, aided by Duke's barber, John Merrick, his butler, W. H. Armstrong, and his cook, Addie Evans, all Negroes, persuaded Washington Duke that a hospital would be a living and more practical memorial. Together with his sons Duke donated a total of $13,000 for the building of Lincoln Hospital at a site on Proctor Street. The details of the gifts, as was customary in the family, were handled by Ben Duke.[31] The city commissioners voted $600 annually for current maintenance; the remainder of the small budget came from private donations. With the building of Lincoln Hospital and a city sewerage system authorized by vote of the people in January, 1901, Durham's health affairs were well provided for except for the lack of a city governmental agency to deal with public health problems. Of the circumstances which made Durham's citizens fear for their health in 1884, only the smell of tobacco dust remained.

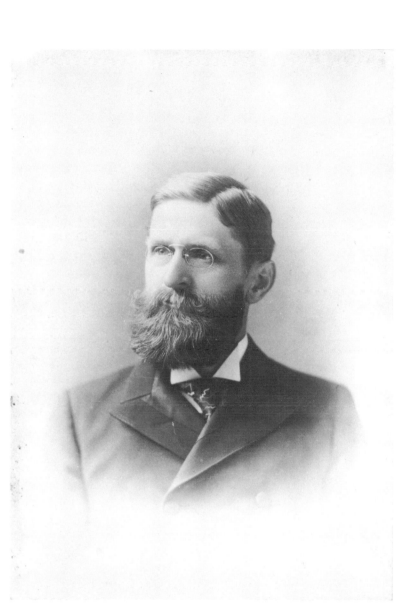

John Franklin Crowell

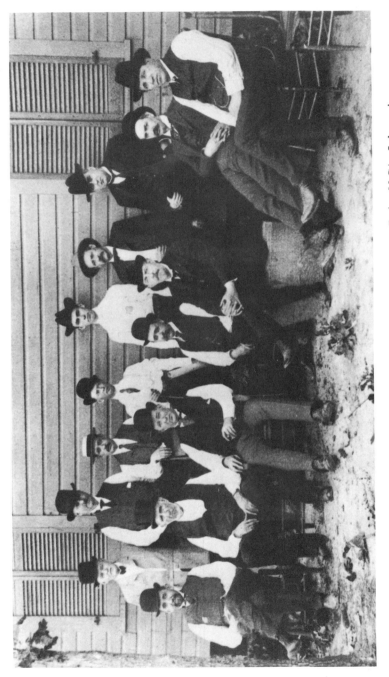

Duke family and business associates, at barbecue in Erwin, N.C. (then known as Duke, N.C.), July or August, 1904. *Front row* (left to right): B. N. Duke, Washington Duke, J. B. Duke, T. J. Walker, A. B. Carrington, J. S. Cobb, John Angier. *Back row* (left to right): Dr. A. G. Carr, W. A. Erwin, J. Ed. Stagg, Frank Tate, E. S. Yarbrough, Capt. Lemon. F. L. Fuller

At the turn of the century both George W. Watts and Ben Duke, on behalf of his family, confined their philanthropy largely to colleges and universities, hospitals, orphanages, and church activities. This policy was prompted by the need for a defense against hundreds of individual requests for aid as well as out of a sense of stewardship of their wealth. Within this pattern each had a favorite philanthropy; Watts the hospital and the Dukes Trinity College.[32] The financial security afforded by the Duke benefactions allowed President Kilgo to publish his version of Trinity's university dream. He was dedicated to quality education under Christian auspices and to the order of priorities set by conditions on Washington Duke's gifts. These were, in order, support of a stronger college faculty, buildings and equipment (particularly library improvements), widening Trinity's constituency without compromising academic standards, and the education of women on an equal basis with men.

Kilgo recognized the need of North Carolina for doctors, and felt that the close proximity of Trinity College and Watts Hospital would make the organization of a two year medical preparatory course an easy matter. He doubted, however, that Durham or any city in North Carolina could furnish the clinical material necessary for a complete medical school. He did propose that Trinity consider establishing courses in pharmacy and a preparatory department in dentistry along with a preclinical medical school but was unwilling to act upon any of these possibilities until a law school was well established at the college. Lawyers, he noted, largely determined lines of legislation and therefore of social development, needed to be guided by the high standards of Christianity, and as a professional group offered the best possibility of extending the patronage of the school.[33] By 1910 Kilgo not only had his law school but also a teacher training program to help meet the demands of North Carolina's new public school system. Moreover, he had also raised faculty salaries. Trinity seemed well on the way to becoming a true university.[34]

The continued success of Duke family businesses made fulfillment of the university dream appear possible. As the Dukes and George Watts diversified their industrial holdings, especially to include textile mills, they became interested in water power as a means of generating electricity to turn the machines in their factories. James B.

Duke was increasingly fascinated by the mechanics of water power after building a power plant on the Raritan River to serve his Somerville, New Jersey farm.[35] In 1905 he organized the Southern Power Company (later Duke Power Company) to develop a unified electric system for the western sections of the Carolinas. It was a bold venture. Only the largest cities enjoyed electric service, furnished, in most instances, by small and insufficient plants. Other mill operators doubted the dependability of electric power, and Duke often was forced to buy stock in his customer's firms to encourage initial investment in electrification. In 1911, when the United States Supreme Court ordered The American Tobacco Company dissolved under anti-trust laws, four power plants were operating and more were under construction. By 1913 Duke directed the investment of some $25,000,000 into water power and related industries; in a few years this sum had doubled. Southern's success insured the continued growth of the Duke family fortune.[36]

Durham grew apace with the success of its tobacco, textile, and related industries. The annexation of the mill towns of East and West Durham placed new demands on the city's public services between 1900 and 1910. All city services were severely taxed, but none more so than the little cottage hospital. Accordingly, in 1909, George Watts again donated a site, money for buildings and equipment, and endowment funds for a new 160-bed hospital at a total cost of over $750,000.[37]

Once again the combination of a larger population, increased local medical needs, and the close proximity of Trinity College to a new hospital resulted in a proposal for a medical school. This time a local physician, Dr. Joseph Graham, attempted to assure the development of such a school by getting advance support for his plan from Watts and B. N. Duke before presenting it to college and hospital officials. He advocated, as had Kilgo, that Trinity College add departments of medicine, dentistry, and pharmacy. The old hospital property, adjacent to the rapidly expanding Trinity campus, would house the new departments under gift from Mr. Watts, and endowment funds would cover expenses over and above income from students.[38]

Watts was agreeable, but B. N. Duke would not be stampeded,

insisting that Graham present his proposals to the Trinity trustees. Standards of medical education had changed considerably since Crowell planned to pay two resident physicians $2000 apiece out of hospital collections and contributions to be the staff of his medical school. The symbol of the new standards was The Johns Hopkins University School of Medicine in Baltimore. There European university practices and an energetic young faculty had placed medical education on a scientific basis. Preclinical students studied in research laboratories rather than lecture rooms, and clinical students learned the art of medicine at bedside conferences in a 225 bed hospital which was an integral part of the university. The professors in the preclinical departments were university teachers paid full salaries to instruct students and pursue research projects, and the pressure of private practice upon the time and energy of the clinical men indicated to some that they too should be freed by university salaries to teach on a full time basis rather than supporting themselves from their practice.[39] These new practices were being adopted by the best medical schools and, everywhere admired, were revolutionizing American ideas about medical education simply by the power of example.

The new concept of basic research as the ground of applied science required expensive laboratory equipment, a large modern hospital, a faculty trained in the most modern methods and a budget adequate to purchase the latest medical knowledge and technology. In the 1880's the Hopkins trustees had refused to develop their medical school with less than half a million dollars in hand.[40] The Trinity trustees for the first time accepted the medical school proposal in principle, but what would it cost? Graham suggested no new sources of endowment. The State Medical Society was still on record as opposed to the use of student fees to pay the salaries of medical school faculty. On motion of C. W. Toms, a former Durham public school administrator made an officer of The American Tobacco Company by James B. Duke, the executive committee of the Trinity trustees approved the addition of schools of medicine, dentistry, and pharmacy to the college, but only if Mr. Watts donated the old hospital for the purpose, if students were given free use of the new Watts hospital, and if an endowment of not less than $300,000 could be raised. Among members of the committee appointed to raise the endowment and develop plans were Dr. Graham, President Kilgo, and the young Dean of Trinity College, William Preston Few.[41]

Son of a physician and graduate of Wofford College and Harvard University, Few had come to Trinity in 1896 to fill a temporary vacancy in the English department. Slight of build, quiet, personable, and industrious, he so impressed Kilgo that the President persuaded B. N. Duke to endow a new chair in English so that Few might be kept at the College.[42] Few apparently decided quickly that Trinity offered him a promising career. Plagued by recurrent eye trouble, he responded warmly to the support of the college community. Writing to Kilgo in 1900, he expressed both his decision and his feelings:

> I can say without a tinge of cant that my chief ambition now is to help in my little way the great work we have begun at the College . . . the treatment I have received during the dark year from the College and from my personal friends in and at the College has bound me to the college with a love that is one of the passions of my life. I hope to spend a good part of my days in attempting to pay the debt of gratitude I owe and I shall be happiest when I am set to do unpleasant tasks for the College.[43]

William Preston Few became Trinity's first dean in 1902. With Kilgo frequently away from the campus speaking to church groups or raising funds, Few gradually assumed responsibility for internal administration, academic affairs, and keeping benefactors of the college informed of progress. In 1903 he was principal author of the statement supporting academic freedom issued by the Trinity trustees when a professor of history, John Spencer Bassett, was attacked by Josephus Daniels, editor of the *Raleigh News and Observer,* for his writings criticizing racism in Democratic party politics. This statement attracted to Trinity and to Few the attention of Wallace Buttrick, President of the General Education Board. This foundation, funded by John D. Rockefeller, promoted improvement of education in the United States, without distinction of race, sex, or creed, particularly in the South where the lowest standards of education in the nation prevailed. This attention was to be important.

When Kilgo was consecrated a bishop of the Methodist Church

in 1910, Few, with the support of Kilgo and Ben Duke, was elected President. The only reservation anyone expressed about his qualifications was that, unlike Kilgo, he was not a great orator. It was feared that Few might not be able to attract funds to the College so successfully as the fiery preacher. Under Kilgo Trinity's endowment had risen from $22,500 to $441,339, and the assets of the College rose from approximately $200,000 to $1,221,382. Trinity, now almost entirely free of financial problems, possessed the largest endowment of any college in the South.[44]

Growing wealth, coupled with articles in Democratic newspapers linking Trinity to the "tobacco trust," made it difficult for the college to obtain funds from philanthropic sources other than the Duke family. Few's success in 1911 in negotiating with Buttrick for a grant of $150,000 towards a million dollar endowment drive established a useful precedent in favor of foundation support of Trinity College, led to close personal contacts between Few and the General Education Board, and brought Few out of the shadow of Kilgo, who still resided on the campus, into his own as a college president.[45] While Few learned the responsibilities of his new position, however, he held the medical school plans in abeyance.

The reluctance of the Trinity trustees to proceed with medical education without substantial endowment was confirmed by the appearance of Abraham Flexner's survey, "Medical Education in the United States and Canada." An avalanche of applications from medical schools for funds to provide newly-important laboratory facilities prompted the Carnegie Foundation to review the quality of education being offered as a guide in funding grant proposals. Flexner measured 155 schools against the standards of admission, size of endowment, training of faculty, access to clinical facilities, and teaching conditions at The Johns Hopkins University School of Medicine. He concluded that the majority of American medical schools were poorly operated commercial ventures turning out ill-trained physicians, and recommended closing all but 31. He could credit North Carolina with a comparatively satisfactory ratio of population to physicians only by counting the unlicensed and unregistered doctors in rural areas. Of the four medical schools in the state, two, the preclinical departments at the University of North Carolina and Wake Forest College, he judged adequate for their purpose. The North Carolina Medical College at Charlotte he condemned as being a stock company in which professorships were bought and sold, income barely maintained the physical plant, entrance requirements were "nominal," and facilities ranged from poor to wretched. The Leonard Medical School in Raleigh, which attempted to train Negro physicians, he found had too little income to succeed.[46]

Flexner's study established the Hopkins model as the standard pattern for American medical schools and completed the revolution started by that school's example and the demands of physicians for tighter medical licensing laws. Whether because of their faults or because Flexner exposed them, dozens of lesser schools closed their doors, among them the four-year schools in Charlotte and Raleigh. Despite Flexner's concern that the state have more trained physicians, North Carolina now lacked a clinical medical school to produce them. Realizing that Trinity could not meet the Hopkins standards set by Flexner, the trustee committee to develop plans for a medical school never officially reported.

Flexner himself left the Carnegie Foundation for the General Education Board when it became clear to him that John D. Rockefeller was more interested than Andrew Carnegie in improving medical education. He was there in 1916 when his brother Simon, a member of the staff of the Rockefeller Institute, showed him a letter from an old friend, William Preston Few.

> An increasing number of graduates of Trinity College are seeking a first-class medical education. For a large number of our graduates the expense of four or five years at a good medical school is well nigh prohibitive. We are being urged over and over again to establish a two-year medical course that would be accepted at good medical schools . . . I should be glad for an expression of your opinion as to the advisability of our undertaking this new line of work, and I should be glad for you to indicate in outline what you think we might undertake to do.[47]

Abraham Flexner and the General Education Board were interested in encouraging medical education in the South and asked immediately for information on Trinity's financial situation. Although Few at this time had no definite plans for a university, he welcomed contact with the General Education Board on matters related to Trinity's support and invited the Board to hold its regional meetings at the College. After 1916 the idea of medicine at Trinity was kept alive before the Board by Abraham Flexner.[48]

America's entry into World War I slowed development at Trinity, however, and no new major projects were started. So far as the medical school idea was concerned, the most important event was the serious illness of Ben Duke in 1917–1918. Confined to a New York hospital, he became despondent. Few, who had had similar experiences and remembered the value of the personal support he received from the college community, wrote Duke a long series of letters which made no requests but which kept him informed about events in Durham, the College, the weather, crops, friends and relatives, and local society. His letters offered Duke continuing reassurance as to the value and importance of his life's work, and cemented what already was a warm friendship between men of similar personalities. Meanwhile in 1918, James B. Duke, who was already hinting to Few that he planned large philanthropies, joined his brother on the Trinity Board of Trustees. "Thus the family ties grew stronger, and the future, though vague, looked promising,"[49] as Few was later to describe the situation.

The end of the war brought increased enrollments and costs both to Trinity and the University of North Carolina. At Chapel Hill Dr. I. H. Manning, dean of the medical school, began to express concern over the large number of students applying for the limited number of places in his department. He noted that the per capita cost of educating students in his small school was rising rapidly and that the school found it difficult to follow the lead of the best medical schools in methods of instruction because of its location (Chapel Hill, like Wake Forest, had a population of fewer than 1500), the scarcity of teachers, and lack of funds. The school, he stated flatly, was not supplying its proper quota of physicians to the state. There were some 400 premed students enrolled in various colleges throughout North Carolina, and the state was expected to issue 100 licenses to practice each year, yet for lack of faculty and equipment he could accept only forty students annually.[50]

This imbalance led Few to reopen discussions with Ben Duke, Abraham Flexner, George Watts, and Watts's son-in-law, John

Sprunt Hill, concerning the possibility of a medical school for Trinity. John D. Rockefeller, encouraged by his son and Flexner, added 45 million dollars to the funds of the General Education Board specifically for the support of medical education, "cooperating with progressive intention wherever found."[51] Regional needs were to be given particular consideration, and no region had more medical needs than the South. The Board was seeking to support a well-organized medical school south of the Potomac River and east of the Appalachians. By this time aware that James B. Duke planned large educational philanthropies, Few was confident that Trinity could meet the matching funds provisions contained in all Rockefeller grants. If the resources of the college could be combined with those of Watts Hospital and the University of North Carolina, Durham was a possible site for such a school.[52]

President Few sought the widest possible cooperation in his new venture. Plans were drawn for a proposal that the federal government locate a Veterans Administration hospital in Durham next to the Watts Hospital site. Through John Sprunt Hill, a trustee of the University of North Carolina, its Board was invited to cooperate, without financial obligation, with a medical college, offering the clinical years of medical instruction only, to be located in a nearby city.[53] Using trade radius maps and census figures he convinced Flexner that there was a sufficient population and communications network within a 200 mile radius of Durham. Crucial months were lost when George Watts died of stomach cancer in the spring of 1921,[54] but his widow wished to continue the project. In June Few shared his hopes for a medical school and the name "university" with the Trinity trustees. The negotiations proceeded slowly, for neither the General Education Board nor Few wished to kill the plan with premature publicity.[55] In December Few outlined his progress and his hopes to C. W. Toms, who often was his confidential mediator in dealing with James Buchanan Duke.

Dr. Flexner and Dr. Buttrick said they thought a medical school here ought to start with $6,000,000 and that they would stand for $3,000,000 of that amount and believed that their local board would, provided we can get another $3,000,000. I told this to Mrs. Watts today, and she said if we could get $2,000,-

ooo of this she thought $1,000,000 could be got here. All of this looks pretty good.

I think you ought to talk to Mr. J. B. D. If he will say he will give us $1,000,000 within five years, I will undertake to raise the rest. If he will give us $2,000,000, success will be assured; and I of course wish he would give three or more.[56]

The delay caused by Watts's death, however, was enough to allow the initiative in developing medical education in the state to pass to the University of North Carolina in Chapel Hill. Under increasing pressure to provide physicians for the state, its medical department found it more and more difficult to transfer its graduates directly into the third year of other medical schools. President H. W. Chase proposed, therefore, an extension of the medical curriculum to four years and the building of the necessary hospital facilities.[57] Governor Cameron Morrison quickly endorsed the proposal. A committee appointed to investigate needs and costs found that the ratio of physicians to population in North Carolina was 1 to 1600 against a recommended level of 1 to 1000, that the ratio of hospital beds to population was 1 to 761 against a national average of 1 to 340, that only four hospitals in North Carolina were recognized for purposes of internship, and that few of North Carolina's hospitals had enough endowment to provide free care for the poor, which reduced the number of patients available for teaching purposes. To build a minimum size modern hospital (200 beds) would cost $750,-ooo and to maintain it would require $250,000 annually. Speaking before the State Medical Association, Manning suggested that these costs could be met by private endowment, municipal funds, or state funds; he favored the latter. He left open the question of whether the hospital should be built at the University or in a city.[58]

For the entire year of 1922 Few was forced to mark time, and to urge the General Education Board to do likewise,[59] while the University trustees moved more rapidly than even President Chase anticipated. A majority of the investigating committee wished the school located in Chapel Hill.[60] The consensus of medical authorities, including Dr. Nathan P. Colwell, Secretary of the Council on Medical Education of the American Medical Association, and Dr. William H. Welch of The Johns Hopkins, was that a four-year school definitely was needed, that it should be under the control of the University, that if at all possible it should be located at the University, and that the opinion of the medical profession of the state should have much weight in any final decisions.[61]

As word of the study spread, however, the civic competition among North Carolina cities emerged once more. The city of Charlotte was particularly anxious to have the school located there, having lost the North Carolina Medical College in 1914. The Mecklenburg County Medical Society, which numbered among its members many graduates of that school, wielded powerful influence with the legislature in Raleigh. The Charlotte Chamber of Commerce produced a detailed brochure setting forth the advantages to a medical school of Charlotte's central location, hospital facilities, comparatively large population, and willingness to contribute to the new school's budget. The brochure alerted national medical authorities to the political controversy surrounding the project and made them reluctant to favor publicly any particular site. Chase claimed the pamphlet cut off his advice from the General Education Board and particularly from Flexner, who refused any involvement in the public controversy.[62] The agitation grew so intense that Governor Morrison feared appropriations for other University projects would be threatened in the economy-minded General Assembly if any location other than Charlotte were chosen. This, as President of the University, Chase could not risk. Neither, however, could he let the matter drop, because the medical practitioners of the state wanted action, the alumni of the University would wonder what happened to the project, and the Charlotte forces would feel that any delay on a decision was a tactic designed to defeat their aspirations.[63]

Few's position now was extremely complicated. He was convinced that the state needed only one good medical school, and was dedicated to the widest possible cooperation to gain it. He had hoped to build it in Durham under Trinity control, using funds from the Duke family and the General Education Board. Cooperation of the Board would insure that the Dukes would not have to bear the whole burden of the medical school and the hospital, and therefore would donate also to the expansion of Trinity's other departments. The Board, however, refused to act until the University plan had been disposed of; Chase also was courting its support. How was Few to preserve the progress he had made toward building a medical school in Durham without coming into conflict with the University, losing the good will of many physicians and perhaps the support of the General Education Board, and risking the possibility that a school built at the University would end all hope for a school at Trinity? In early December he wrote to Ben Duke, urgently suggesting a conference with James Buchanan Duke to decide what they would do.

> I still believe if you and Mr. J. B. wish it we can get this medical school; or through the Rockefeller Board we can have some part in its control; and if we should completely fail I feel sure that we can handle the matter in such a way as to leave the College stronger in the eyes of the Rockefeller people and other such great foundations. . . . Whatever is done must be done within the next few weeks.[64]

Few's solution emerged at a meeting of the University of North Carolina Board of Trustees on December 20, 1922, at which the committee investigating the medical school was to make its final report. Knowing that any report he could make for the University alone would kill all hope for a medical school, President Chase presented instead, with the endorsement of Governor Morrison, a proposal by Few that the University and Trinity cooperate in the building of a medical school located at Durham which could serve the purposes of both institutions. Wake Forest College and Davidson College were also invited to participate. The proposed school would be constructed with funds from a $4,000,000 bond issue by the state and an equal amount to be raised by Few from other sources. Control would be vested in a board of trustees on which the two schools would be equally represented. Watts Hospital would be open for teaching purposes.[65] On the same day Few wrote to both Flexner and Ben Duke. He reported Chase, Governor Morrison, "and every other thoughtful man I talked with" enthusiastic, and expected agreement all along the line if a sound plan could be agreed upon, predicted opposition from Josephus Daniels's *Raleigh News and Observer* and "a good deal of splashing of the waters" at the lower levels of power.[66]

The plan exploded in the press, and Few proved an accurate prophet. He was variously reported to have millions of dollars in hand and to be unsure of any support at all. He feared that what he called "the atmosphere of floating millions" would offend James B. Duke and the General Education Board, and kept busy making public and private disavowals of published figures. From Raleigh Josephus Daniels observed an almost unanimous sentiment among the Baptists of North Carolina against any institutional union of church and state, and his paper predicted that the venture would fail. As a University trustee he favored a medical school exclusively controlled by the University. Some Trinity alumni believed that Trinity alone should control the school. The Baptist opposition and the continuing competition among the cities to have the school located within their boundaries, however, seemed to make unified control of the project impossible.[67]

Eugene Clyde Brooks, former Trinity professor who in his position as State Superintendent of Public Instruction acted as liaison between Few and Chase, proposed that Few try to save the project by agreeing that the President of the University be, ex officio, president of the trustees of the medical school. Chase himself, however, was now opposed to any form of control other than complete University control, and so advised Governor Morrison.[68] Knowing this, Few told B. N. Duke:

> I have become convinced that the plan I have been working on for a medical school here will not get through the present Legislature for two reasons: (1) President Chase's crowd has gone back on him, and (2) as things stand now all those who have made askings of this Legislature are going to have all they can do to get what they consider as their necessary appropriations. . . .[69]

When the University trustees announced the decision to build their own medical school on January 25, competing bids for the school came from Raleigh, Greensboro, Durham, Charlotte, Asheville, and Chapel Hill. John Sprunt Hill, who led the Durham delegation before the University trustees, had Few's nominal support in seeking the school for Durham. After all presentations were made, the University trustees resolved to recommend to the General Assembly the building of a four-year school, but no location was mentioned. The suggested appropriation was made so small as to indicate that the University placed a low priority on the project, and when the request was not pushed, the Legislature made no appropriation at all. The proposal finally was referred for study to the Council on Medical Education of the American Medical Association.[70] All parties to the discussion, however, expressed gratitude to Few for his efforts to reconcile the opposing interests.

With the fate of his second cooperative plan no longer in doubt, Few sent parallel letters to Abraham Flexner and B. N. Duke. To both he recounted the reasons for the project's failure; to Flexner he spoke of the continuing need for the school; to Duke he suggested that "we may even yet get from outside sources a considerable amount of money for a medical school to belong wholly to us."[71] To C. W. Toms, however, he expressed his fear that the University might well "come to Durham with its medical school and have the cooperation of the hospitals here which by right belong first to us and get money from the outside at which we had the first chance." He implored Toms to find out what definite decisions James B. Duke had made concerning Trinity. In March Few met with Duke himself to discuss those decisions, and reported to Toms that "Mr. Duke wished especially to see me about our proposed medical school and a strong silent movement to take it to Charlotte. The latter will of course never come to pass, but the medical school is now in shape when I believe I can carry it through, if we can without delay provide for the development of our enlarged institution."[72]

In order to forestall any action by the University that would threaten his new plans, Few wrote on the same day to Dr. J. W. Long, President of the State Medical Society, telling him unofficially that he could safely asume that Trinity would build a medical school and without too much delay.[73] Dean Manning appeared before the Society in April to plead the University's case. The discussion of the cooperative plan had proved the need for a medical school, he felt, and the location of a medical school on a university campus was an "American ideal."[74] The University's drive to secure the support of the Society, however, was blunted by lack of definite plans, unified alumni support, and funds for building a medical school. When the final report of the Society's Committee to Consider the Four Year Medical School was delivered the following year, the mood of the state's physicians became crystal clear. Dr. I. W. Faison, then 71, former dean and professor of pediatrics of the North Carolina Medical College and the most influential of Charlotte physicians who had fought to have the proposed medical school located in their city,[75] spoke for the committee: "I want a school. I want it located at the place best suited for a great school, equipped and manned by men, even paid men, by the state, who can cope with men in any school, and who can and will draw men from other states. My time in life forbids me to allow my optimism to hope for this, still I shall hope."[76]

By accepting Faison's report the doctors of North Carolina declared that old loyalties no longer would stand in the way of building a four-year medical school, whatever the location, which met the standards first set at The Johns Hopkins and made normative by Flexner's 1910 survey. Few now was confident that the resources needed to meet these standards soon would be available to Trinity. The failure of his cooperative plan, he felt, "served two good purposes—it kept the road open for a first-rate School of Medicine later on, and it put Mr. James B. Duke on his mettle."[77]

Chapter 3: Natural Resources Supporting Social Services: The Duke Endowment, 1923–1927

As early as 1916, James B. Duke told William Preston Few of his intention to give away, during his lifetime, a large part of his fortune. He hoped to include in this his electric power holdings but only if these were in a position to pay dividends.[1] His philosophy was to arrange his philanthropy so that the profits from the natural water resources of the Carolinas were directed to the social needs of their residents.[2] As he planned his gifts, the last of his major investments, a series of electric power plants in Canada, paid off through a union with The Aluminum Company of America. This potentially lucrative merger assured ample funds for expanding Trinity College into Duke University, to include both a medical school and hospital, as well as for Mr. Duke's other charitable projects. Mr. Duke's unexpected death in 1925, however, left William Preston Few with three unrelated problems: how to protect as much of Duke's legacy as possible for charitable purposes, how to keep other foundations interested in supporting the new and apparently wealthy university, and how to select the man to have charge of the university's largest single component, the medical division.

James B. Duke was a public figure but a private man. He never made speeches, rarely issued public statements, and only occasionally granted to anyone outside his circle of business associates the kind of interview that might illuminate his motivations. His few personal papers were destroyed, and consequently his biographers have turned largely to anecdotes to explain his intentions, particularly with reference to his gifts to medicine.[3] The lessons of his life better explain, however, why the "tough-minded, ambitious man of property, indifferent to theory and abstraction, dedicated, rather, to putting to use his gift of discerning how material progress can be made to happen"[4] became the patron of medical care throughout North and South Carolina.

Among his continuing experiences were three which moved Mr. Duke to include medicine among the primary objects of his philanthropy. The earliest of these influences was the pattern of giving he shared with his father and brother. "If I amount to anything in this world," Duke was fond of repeating, "I owe it to my daddy and the Methodist Church."[5] Though this statement has been overworked by biographers, there is no reason to doubt its authenticity. Washington Duke, as we have seen, made substantial contributions to hospitals, as well as to colleges, orphanages, and the Methodist Church, and his sons had shared in these projects. As late as 1924 James B. Duke and his brother, Ben, contributed $75,000 toward the cost of rebuilding Lincoln Hospital in Durham.[6] Winkler has suggested that Duke's gifts to medicine reflected a desire to emulate the giving of others, especially the senior Rockefeller.[7] Certainly Duke was not unaware of Rockefeller's giving, nor of those of other philanthropists, but this awareness is best understood as supporting a long-established habit of giving by the Duke family.

In 1914 James B. Duke united this family practice with his proposals for the disposal of his personal fortune. His success in tobacco manufacturing was based upon selling to the average man. His success in the electric power industry grew out of his vision of a series of connected power houses pouring a steady stream of energy to a multitude of users. He extended this vision into a plan to give this power system to the communities it served in such a manner that they could finance their own charities simply by doing business in the usual way.[8] Among the needs of the people was adequate health care. As he characteristically put it, "without good doctors they cannot live."[9]

From 1916, when Duke first intimated his intention to develop Trinity College into a university as a part of his philanthropy, William Preston Few, patiently but persistently, pressed him with the idea of building a medical school and hospital that would serve the state both as a referral center and a source of trained medical personnel. When Duke was ready to decide how his funds should be apportioned, Few presented for his consideration the following outline plan of a new university which included provision for a medical school:

I [James B. Duke] wish to see Trinity College, the law school & other schools expanded into a fully developed university organization. It has been suggested to me that this expanded institution be named Duke University as a memorial to my father

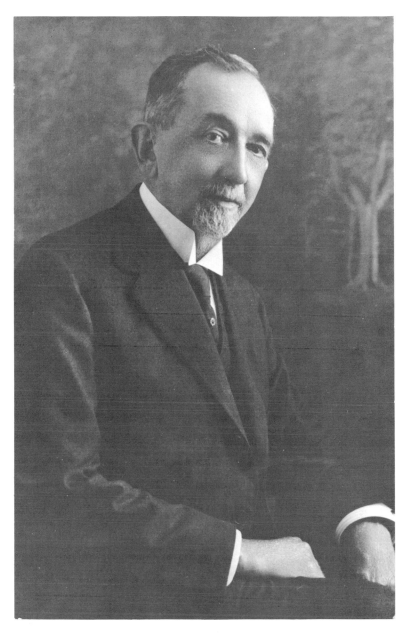

B. N. Duke

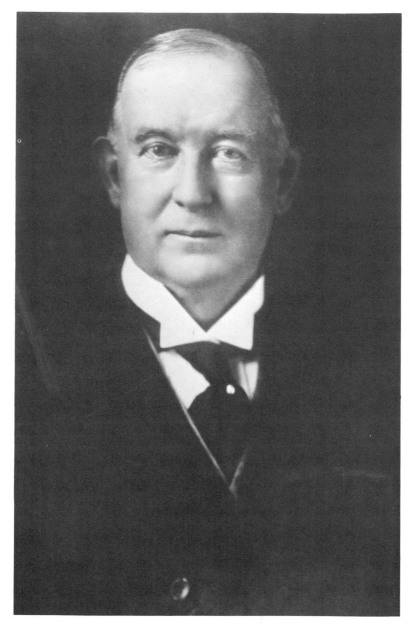

James Buchanan Duke

[Washington Duke] whose gifts made possible the building of Trinity College in Durham, and I approve this suggestion. I desire this university to include Trinity College, a coordinate College for Women, a Law School, a School of Religious Training, a School of Education, a School of Business Administration, a School of Engineering (emphasizing chemical & electrical engineering), a Graduate School of Arts & Sciences, and, when adequate funds are available, a Medical School. I desire this enlarged institution to be operated under the present charter with only such changes, if any changes at all, as this enlargement may require. To this university that is to be thus organized I will give —— millions of dollars. I agree to pay in within —— years —— millions either in cash or good securities.[10]

In 1923, with his power holdings in the Carolinas well established and producing dividends, Duke placed his secretary, Alexander H. Sands, Jr., in charge of surveying the health care needs of the Carolinas.[11] National surveys indicated that both North and South Carolina were short of physicians. North Carolina had one doctor for every 1150 residents and South Carolina one for every 1231 as compared to a national average of 1 to 724.[12] North Carolina had, in relation to its area, a smaller number of places having physicians than any other state of comparable population density. In both states the shortage was increasingly acute in rural areas, from which doctors, especially the younger men, tended to migrate to the cities.[13] Hospital beds were in similarly short supply.

Duke asked Sands to make a complete survey of the number and location of hospitals in the Carolinas, how they were controlled, the number of free and pay beds they operated, the percentage of their charges they collected from patients, and the net cost of the charity care they provided, as the basis for devising a philanthropic formula which would help to provide both doctors and hospitals in the medically underdeveloped areas of the two states. Sands asked Few to assist him in collecting the data,[14] and Few in turn consulted Dr. Watson S. Rankin, Secretary of the State Board of Health, who had vigorously supported Few's cooperative medical school plan the preceding year.[15] Together they considered not only Duke's plans for hospitals in the Carolinas but also how these plans could be related to Few's desire for a hospital and medical school at Trinity that would serve as a referral center for the entire state.[16]

At Few's suggestion Rankin drafted a memo for presentation to Duke outlining their conclusions. The plan was based upon the premise that Trinity would administer the funds available to other hospitals through the proposed Duke foundation. The central hospital would serve also as a collection and evaluation agency for the records of local hospitals, as an advising agency in matters of administration and management, as a referral center in medical matters, and as a teaching center for the state's medical profession, providing postgraduate courses during the summer months. A similar system, Rankin suggested, might be arranged in South Carolina.[17]

Sands also consulted directly with Rankin as to how general hospitals could be developed in North Carolina. At Sands's request, Rankin developed his ideas in more detail. His model was a plan developed by Dr. M. M. Seymour, a health officer in Saskatchewan, Canada, for use in that province.[18] Discoveries in bacteriology, chemistry, physics and instrumentation, he wrote, had forced modern medicine to become institutionalized. Successful practice was impossible without the ward and laboratory training, complex equipment, and group practice arrangements afforded by a hospital. As a result, physicians crowded into cities, where such facilities were available, and rural areas were denuded of doctors. Much of North Carolina, being rural, was in this situation. To reverse this flight, hospitals had to be built in the rural areas. The cost for construction and maintenance of such hospitals was beyond the intelligent appreciation of the average rural voter or taxpayer, hence hospitals could not be supported solely by local tax funds. Yet it was important that outside help not substitute for but stimulate local self-help, for health care was properly a community responsibility.

Rankin suggested aiding counties or communities willing to assume the cost of building a hospital (approximately $100,000 for fifty beds) by having a portion of the maintenance cost (estimated at $3.00 per bed per day) subsidized, especially in instances where the hospitals set aside a percentage of their bed capacity for charity care. He advocated placing control of such hospitals with the local community, so as to insure responsible and increasing community support for the hospital. He also advised requiring hospitals receiving aid to keep records which could be compared with those of other hospitals as a check on costs, methods, and results. The trustees of the foundation then would be in a position to advise helpfully in the organization and management of the local hospitals, study state-wide needs, carry on public education activities, encourage legisla-tive support of hospitals, provide a visiting consultant service, and supply teams of nurses and technicians for teaching local workers the technical methods involved in their specialties and needed in the rural community. When Sands explained that improving medical care in the Carolinas was only one of James B. Duke's philanthropic proposals and that all would be administered by a foundation related directly to the power company, Rankin dropped the idea of handling hospital funds through Trinity College.[19]

At the same time Mr. Duke's plans for expanding Trinity College into a new university advanced to the building stage. With his architect, Horace Trumbauer of Philadelphia, he surveyed the cam-pus and approved Trumbauer's sketches of stone buildings of Gothic architecture. Under Few as president the top levels of the new uni-versity's administration took shape, with Robert L. Flowers in charge of business operations and William H. Wannamaker, for many years Few's advisor on curriculum, in charge of educational affairs. During October and November, in consultation with officials of the Rocke-feller foundations, Mr. Duke planned the financial structure of the university and its relation to his own foundation. Few's suggestion that the Trinity College trustees administer the foundation was abandoned since the foundation trustees were to be charged with operating the Duke Power Company. A separate board would pro-vide the business experience and talent necessary for operating a public utility without placing university trustees in the power busi-ness.[20]

At the same time, the climax of a long series of events substantially increased the potential worth of the new foundation.[21] In developing the Southern Power Company, as his combine was then called, Duke had continually faced the problem of disposing of the excess generat-ing capacity of his plants. On trips to Europe he secured rights to processes for fixation of nitrogen and manufacture of chemical fertilizers in hopes of selling power, indirectly, to the tobacco in-dustry in the Carolinas.

Always a man of large vision, Duke began to consider sites outside the Carolinas for his nitrogen plant and associated power development. The Aluminum Company of America, faced with an increasing shortage of power sources, asked Duke to consider building his plant in Canada and sharing the energy with the aluminum industry. While on a trip to inspect possible sites for power stations in Seattle, Washington, and Canada, Duke met by chance Thomas L. "Carbide" Willson, the first man to secure a grant for electric power development in Canada from the British crown. Willson showed Duke the gorges of the Saugenay River. Duke, impressed, bought rights on the river and began to build power stations there in 1914. Immediately, however, he again faced the problem of excess capacity. Electric power was being replaced by purely chemical processes for fixing nitrogen, and with no other customers for his power immediately available, Duke stopped work on his Canadian plants.

In 1920, however, a great increase in the number of magazines and periodicals in America created a heavy demand for newsprint which in turn brought a demand by newsprint producers, notably Sir William Price of Price Brothers and Company, Limited, for electric power. Duke's Quebec Development Company, in which Price became a minority stockholder, began building a large power plant on the Saugenay at Isle Maligne. Duke's plans called for a plant producing far more electric power than the newsprint industry needed, so the search for customers began anew.

One of the few potential buyers was George D. Hoskell of Springfield, Massachusetts, who asked to reserve 50,000 horsepower for his Bausch Machine Tool Company, a small producer of aluminum sheets. Although Duke quickly determined that this company was too small to be an important customer, the Hoskell request set him to investigating whether aluminum could be better produced in the Saugenay region than elsewhere. With the opening of his Isle Maligne station fast approaching, Duke approached Arthur Vining Davis of The Aluminum Company of America with the idea of building an aluminum smelter near Isle Maligne to take 50,000 to 100,000 horsepower. The large amount of readily available power, low development costs in the area, and ease of access to ocean navigation made the project a natural for the aluminum producer. These successful negotiations led to plans for Duke to develop a second power site on the Saugenay, Chute á Caron, to be merged with The Aluminum Company of America in return for a one-ninth interest in the company, valued then at approximately seventeen million dollars.

Buoyed by the knowledge that his long-disappointing Canadian power investments were about to yield large dividends, Mr. Duke arrived in Charlotte with his personal counsel, William R. Perkins, on December 1, 1924. They were joined by Duke business associates Anthony J. D. Biddle, Jr., George G. Allen, Norman A. Cocke, C. F. Burkholder, E. C. Marshall and Charlotte attorney E. T. Cansler. At 8:30 that Monday morning Mr. Duke announced to the group that he had been planning for some years to create an educational and charitable foundation and that the group would stay assembled until the job was completed. Perkins had compiled data and prepared drafts of a proposed charter for the new foundation; each section was discussed by the group. While others worked on the sections, Mr. Duke, under Perkins's guidance, drew up his will, although he did not show it to his other advisors. By Thursday both documents were finished,[22] the charter ready for immediate publication.

On December 11, 1924, Duke made his designs public. An indenture of trust created a perpetual foundation, The Duke Endowment. The beneficiaries, including orphanages, hospitals, educational institutions, and the Methodist Church, were those which the Duke family had supported for decades. He turned over to The Endowment securities valued at approximately $40,000,000, with the income to be distributed as stated in the indenture. Twenty percent was to be set aside until another $40,000,000 had accumulated. Of the remaining net income, Trinity College received 32 percent if and when it changed its name to Duke University. Few's plan for a university was included almost verbatim. Mr. Duke envisioned Trinity College as the undergraduate college for men in the new university. He suggested adding to it a coordinate college for women and graduate schools of religion, education, chemistry, law, medicine, business administration, arts and sciences and engineering. The Endowment trustees were instructed to provide $6,000,000 for building the university, once the name was changed, and Duke added a gift of $2,000,000 for this purpose. Davidson College and Furman University each received 5 percent and Johnson C. Smith University, a school for Negroes in Charlotte, 4 percent.

Thirty-two percent was set aside for the support of every hospital in the Carolinas not operated for private gain, according to a formula based upon Sands's research and Rankin's recommendations. Each hospital was allotted up to one dollar per day for every day of care given to charity patients. Any funds remaining under this provision after each hospital received its funds were earmarked for constructing or equipping new hospitals. In explaining this provision Mr. Duke stated that he deemed the need of adequate health care so urgent that he wished every community would assure its residents adequate hospital facilities.

Twelve percent of the income from the new foundation was designated for the Methodist Church, 10 percent for building and maintaining rural churches and 2 percent for the support of retired Methodist preachers. Ten percent was given for the support of orphans, white and Negro, in the Carolinas. The trustees of The Endowment received a fixed percentage of the annual income of the foundation as payment for their services.[23]

President Few encountered no legal difficulties in changing Trinity College into Duke University. The Trinity trustees readily approved the change of name and insertion of the words that the institution "shall have perpetual existence" in the college charter. Administratively, of course, Few's difficulty was only beginning. Letters from alumni protesting the change of name, from job seekers, from suppliants seeking funds for a wide variety of projects, flooded his desk. Even the patient Few became exasperated. To an alumnus who insisted that the new university should be located in Asheville, Few replied that Mr. Duke disapproved of the idea. "When you go out to get $40,000,000 from a man," he added, "you will find that he has some ideas of his own."[24] There were more serious questions, however, about the structure of the university's government. Leading educators opposed the power of the Methodist Church to confirm trustees. Educators and foundations alike asked who controlled the University, the University or the Endowment trustees? Some questioned the fitness of the Trinity College trustees and administrators alike for so large an undertaking. Finally, there was a widespread opinion that the University did not have sufficient funds to accomplish its goals. Few agreed, noting, however, that University policy was to undertake only projects for which funds were at hand.[25]

No project provoked more questions than the anticipated medical school. Under Item VIII of Mr. Duke's will he had provided for ten million dollars to be given to The Duke Endowment, of which four million were to be expected as soon as the Endowment trustees thought reasonable in erecting and equipping a medical school, hospital, and nurses home at Duke University, with the income from the remainder to go to the University.[26] Under Item XI he bequeathed 90 percent of his residuary estate, which probably amounted to as much as the original $40,000,000, to the hospitalization section of The Duke Endowment.[27] Duke did not make these designs public, however, preferring to watch developments in Canada a bit longer. If Few knew of these provisions, and he must have, he kept them secret. To one correspondent who petitioned for the building of a nursing school at Duke he replied only that a nursing school would be a part of any medical school built at Duke.[28] Increasingly he was embarrassed by news stories anticipating developments at Duke, and felt forced to promise in print that he would release all such information at the proper time.[29] For the time being he had to be content with supervising the construction of eleven new buildings on the old Trinity campus.[30]

Mr. Duke himself was slightly less reticent, confiding to friends his dream for the best medical center between Baltimore and New Orleans.[31] He would not, however, live to see it. In the summer of 1925 Duke suffered an almost complete physical breakdown and a gradual wasting which physicians diagnosed as pernicious anemia. On October 10, 1925, he died.[32]

Public reaction to Mr. Duke's provision for a medical school and hospital was overwhelmingly favorable once the terms of his will were known.[33] The project was immediately threatened by provisions of the Revenue Act of 1924, however. Under a complicated formula for taxing large estates earmarked only in part for charitable purposes, the federal government might claim up to eight million dollars and reduce the income of The Duke Endowment by $400,000 annually.[34] The then pending Revenue Act of 1926 changed the formula considerably to the advantage of such estates, but Few, Duke's executors, and apparently some congressmen feared that to apply for retroactive relief would seem to the public an appeal for special favors to big business. Despite an appeal from Representative R. L. Doughton of North Carolina, the bill passed the House with no relief provisions. In the Senate, however, North Carolina's Furnifold M. Simmons held an influential position on the Finance Committee. At his suggestion Few appealed to businessmen, lawyers, public officials, educators and pastors throughout the South to write their congressmen and senators favoring relief. With this support Simmons finally did succeed in persuading the Finance Committee to reduce the basic rate of taxation by half and to eliminate the formula which increased the tax on estates only partially earmarked for charity. On February 19, 1926, a House-Senate conference committee concurred on the new Revenue Act with this amendment intact.[35]

President Few now faced the opposite problem; how to win the support of other major benefactors for Duke University despite its appearance of wealth. The specific bequest for the medical school and hospital was amply secured by 51,236 shares of preferred stock in The Aluminum Company of America.[36] The Endowment trustees were anxious to discharge their responsibilities under the will, and authorized Horace Trumbauer to prepare preliminary sketches of a medical school, hospital, and nurses home.[37] Few would have preferred to move slowly. In the long-standing interest of the General Education Board in the medical development of the South lay his best chance of securing major outside funds, establishing the precedent for foundation giving to Duke University, and quashing public criticism that Duke was attempting too much.[38]

Few also needed the Board's advice in the selection of a dean for the medical school, and with construction soon to start the choice could not be long delayed. As a matter of policy Few delegated full authority in each University department to its administrative head. Since the medical department would be the largest in the University, he had to seek the best and fullest possible advice. Accordingly he reopened contact both with Wallace Buttrick and with Dr. Wycliffe Rose, who was heading up the Rockefeller-financed campaign against hookworm disease in North Carolina. Through Rose he approached Dr. William H. Welch, professor of pathology at The Johns Hopkins University School of Medicine and recognized dean of American medicine, for help in locating "the best man available to take charge of the medical plans, election of faculty, etc."[39] At a Baltimore dinner in March, 1926, Few met for the first time Welch's choice for the post, then Assistant Dean of The Johns Hopkins University School of Medicine, pediatrician Wilburt Cornell Davison.[40]

Davison immediately was Few's first choice, but not his first priority. Having started to recruit a medical school faculty, he now had to involve the General Education Board directly in his plans or lose all hope of their financial support. Recalling to Flexner how together they had struggled to bring a medical school to the Carolinas, Few sought a contribution of $4,000,000 from the Board to the endowment of the medical school and hospital.[41] Such a grant, he argued, would assure the adequate endowment of the other departments of the University and thereby strengthen the entire institution. The Board demurred. Their policy was to support only one school in a region, and in 1923 they had committed themselves to strengthening the medical school at Vanderbilt University to give leadership to Southern medicine. James B. Duke's will seemed to direct $6,000,-000 directly to the endowment of the medical school and hospital. Why, they asked, was more money necessary? Most important, however, the question of control of the medical school was not clear. The Board did not wish large involvement in a school where the trustees of The Duke Endowment might coerce additional funds from the Board by cutting off their own support of the school.[42]

Few delayed for months before proceeding with plans for the medical school, using his reputation for proceeding carefully in all matters to buy time. He carefully scrutinized every available publication by Davison and by another candidate for a medical school appointment, Dr. Harold L. Amoss. He wrote to national medical authorities asking for evaluations of other possible candidates for the deanship.[43] Pressure for action came from all sides. Reports from Dr. Beaumont Cornell, whose search for a cure for pernicious anemia was supported by a grant from Duke University, spoke highly of Dr. Davison. Few could not forever withhold a decision on the deanship.[44] Newspaper accounts of construction plans increased local interest.[45] In November both Davison and Rankin presented papers to the Southern Medical Association, meeting in Atlanta. Davison, Rankin reported, was completely in agreement with the program of the Hospital Section of The Duke Endowment to attract physicians to rural areas by assisting local communities to build hospitals and to insure their efficient operation by regular analysis of their medical and administrative affairs. Although he responded only that he was pleased to know Davison was a good possibility, Few realized that the time he had allotted for gaining additional endowment funds was running out.[46]

In January Few made final the decision he had postponed almost a year. After explaining his plans for development of the medical school to Welch and Lewis H. Weed, Dean of The Johns Hopkins University School of Medicine, he and Davison met and agreed on a salary, $11,000 per year. Few was disappointed by the failure of the General Education Board to renew their earlier support of his efforts; Davison was delighted to begin planning the new medical school free of obligation to old concepts. On January 21, an exchange of telegrams confirmed the appointment and served as a contract.[47]

You have been elected. Delighted with prospect of working with you.
    —W. P. Few

Delighted with honor. Wish to express to you my great appreciation.
    —W. C. Davison[48]

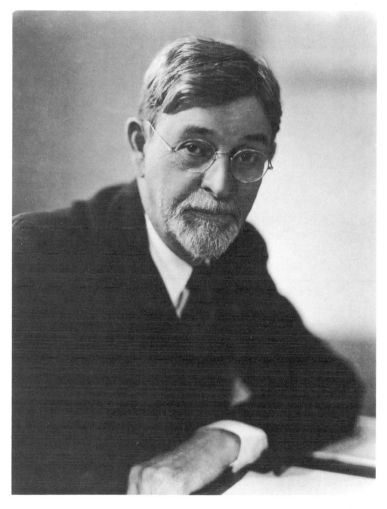

William Preston Few

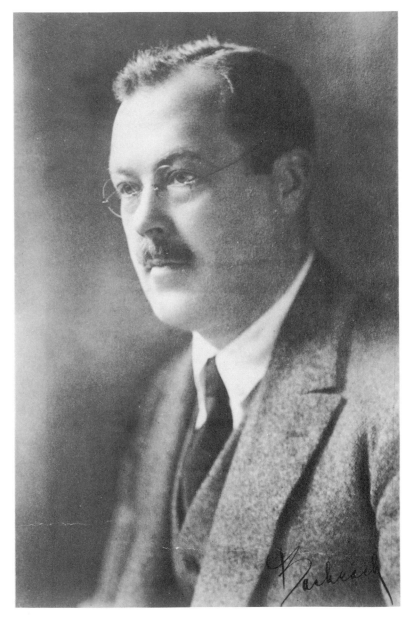

Wilbert C. Davison

Chapter 4: Imprint of an Education: The Building, 1927–1931

Wilburt Cornell Davison developed the philosophy and the priorities which governed the building of the Duke University School of Medicine and Hospital out of his knowledge of medical history and the unique experience of an unorthodox medical education and an early administrative career. Each of his major methods, recruiting a young but able faculty, liberalizing the medical curriculum, and proposing that people pay for medical care through some variant of the insurance principle, was individually justified by historical precedent. Davison's contribution lay in combining his own experience, James B. Duke's legacy, and the lessons of the Hopkins-led American medical revolution into a unified plan which promised to realize Duke's twin objectives: to achieve recognizable excellence quickly and to cooperate with The Duke Endowment in raising the standards of medical care throughout the Carolinas.

Wilburt Cornell Davison was born in Grand Rapids, Michigan, on April 28, 1892, but spent most of his childhood in various towns on Long Island, New York. As the son of a Methodist minister, he endured a series of moves from parish to parish, acquiring from the experience at least one asset—the ability to recognize and call by name the literally hundreds of persons who at any one time made up the current congregation. His father was also a firm believer in rigorous academic discipline. When young Davison was injured playing football and had to stay out of school for the remainder of the year, his father hired a Harvard graduate to teach him Latin and Greek. Six hours of assigned reading and two hours of quizzing six days a week developed a real appreciation for the meaning of hard work. He entered Princeton University in 1909. There, in addition to earning membership in Phi Beta Kappa while active in crew and water polo, he won in 1913 a Rhodes Scholarship for study at Oxford University.[1]

Davison sailed for England in the last week of September, 1913, to enter Merton College, Oxford. Using a catalogue from The Johns Hopkins University Medical School as his guide, he outlined for his first year a course of study covering the first two years of The Hopkins curriculum and obtained permission to follow this program from Sir William Osler, the Regius Professor of Medicine and dean of the medical school. Osler and the young American quickly became friends; during his first year Davison not only attended Osler's weekly ward rounds at Radcliffe Infirmary but also was invited to informal seminars on the history of medicine at Sir William's home. Davison relied on his distinguished mentor's influence to open the doors of leading schools and clinics for further study: anatomy at the University of Edinburgh, surgery at Sir Arbuthnot Lane's clinic at Guy's Hospital, London, and obstetrics at the Rotunda Hospital in Dublin.[2]

When the British medical schools closed upon the outbreak of war in Europe, Davison was one of the many American students who volunteered to serve with the French army. He was assigned to a military hospital outside of Paris, where, because of the brevity of his medical education, he served first as an orderly, later as an anesthetist. In part to escape these rather menial duties, he volunteered in January, 1915, to join an expedition to Serbia to fight an epidemic of typhus. There was no specific treatment, and Davison's patients died like flies in the small, mud-walled, overcrowded, lice-infested hovels of the towns of Krusevar and Nis. Three of the Americans serving in Serbia died of the disease. Only by strict enforcement of sanitary measures could the epidemic even be controlled, yet local officials would not allow the draining of surface water or the breaking of windows to air the mud houses for fear of irritating the fatalistic populace. The experience left Davison with a vivid awareness of the necessity of basic health care for all people.[3]

After two and a half months in Serbia, Davison made his way back across Europe to England, arriving late in April. As the war dragged on the British medical schools had reopened, and Davison resumed his studies under Osler's guidance. At the suggestion of Sir William he investigated the efficacy of triple typhoid-paratyphoid vaccine by agglutination tests on rabbits and fellow medical students, under the supervision of Osler and Georges Dreyer, professor of pathology. The results of these experiments, which helped to justify the adoption of the vaccine by the British Army, became the basis of Davison's first scholarly publication. This paper later caught the attention of the National Research Council in the United States when the American Expeditionary Force considered adopting the triple vaccine. Also, as Osler's intern, he compiled case histories, administered anesthetics, assisted at operations, and wrote up case notes for Osler and other senior staff members. In 1915 he took a B.A. at Oxford, and in 1916 a B.Sc.[4]

By the summer of 1916, however, it became obvious that America soon would enter the war. With Osler's recommendation he was given credit for the first three years of the normal medical school curriculum and returned home to enter the senior class at The Johns Hopkins University School of Medicine. His unique experience had convinced him that medical students should take an active part in planning their course of studies in accord with their personal interests, that research should be a major part of the student's curriculum, and that for learning the art of medicine there was no substitute for close personal contact with professors. After the exciting pace at Oxford, Davison at first found The Hopkins dull. His research work was ended, at least for a time, and his patient load had abruptly dropped from over a hundred to five or six. Soon, however, attending clinics under John Howland, pediatrician-in-chief at The Hopkins, rekindled an interest first awakened by watching Osler at work on the children's wards of the Radcliffe Infirmary, and Davison decided to become a pediatrician. Under the sting of Howland's remorseless criticism Davison relearned the basic lessons imparted by the quiet and self-effacing Osler: the necessity of a long work day, the importance of keeping abreast of medical journals, ward rounds as the basis of medical teaching, and the value of chemical procedures as aids to diagnosis.[5]

When the United States at last formally declared war on April 6, 1917, Davison promptly secured an early graduation from The Hopkins and an assignment in U.S. Army Field Hospital No. 1, which had been earmarked for overseas duty. Davison's army laboratory work was enlivened by visits three times a week to a war orphanage where he was able to put his training in pediatrics to good use. After the Armistice and a few months in charge of the laboratory work at Base Hospital 33 in Portsmouth, England, he returned to the United States in February, 1919, having arranged with Howland for a position at Harriet Lane, children's clinic of The Johns Hopkins University Hospital.[6]

From 1919 to 1927 Davison held teaching and administrative positions in the Department of Pediatrics at The Hopkins. During these years he published 36 papers and two books. The earliest of these were studies in clinical and laboratory pediatrics. After 1925, however, when at Howland's instigation he was appointed assistant to Dean Lewis H. Weed at The Hopkins, his writings began to reflect administrative concerns such as the construction of the curriculum and the selection of medical students. These articles attracted the attention of national medical authorities and were the basis of the favorable recommendations Few received on Davison when he solicited suggestions for the Duke deanship prior to his first meeting with Welch. This administrative experience, and the personal example of the benign dictator, Howland, were at the heart of the philosophy of medical education and administration which Davison brought to Duke in 1927. Harvard surgeon Harvey Cushing, who knew both Davison and the job he was tackling, wrote, "Congratulations on your Dukedom. Much power to your elbow."[7]

Reaction to Davison's appointment was overwhelmingly favorable.[8] For Davison, however, there was work to be done even before the congratulations were in. Architect Horace Trumbauer's initial plans for the new medical school and hospital were already drawn up, and the Endowment trustees were anxious to begin construction. Both the Tudor Gothic style of the buildings and the multicolored stone for the walls had been selected long since by Trumbauer and James B. Duke, but within the walls it was necessary to arrange the location of the various clinical and preclinical departments, administrative offices, and service areas for maximum efficiency of operation. For help on this problem Trumbauer secured the services of Winford H. Smith, Director of The Johns Hopkins Hospital, as consulting medical architect.[9] Davison and Smith agreed to follow the pattern of the Vanderbilt, Chicago, and Rochester schools by relating the departments to each other within the building according to their relationship in practice. Thus, for example, the surgery and pathology departments were closely associated, and the x-ray department was placed as nearly as possible equidistant from medicine, surgery, and the out-patient department.[10]

In the months before he was to go to Durham, while the land for the new campus was being leveled by mules and draglines and a

railroad spur built to the site to haul steel and stone for the buildings, Davison set out to learn as much as possible about medicine in
North Carolina and to publicize his plans for medicine at Duke.
Those plans were threatened by the final decision of the General
Education Board not to participate in raising new endowment funds
for the University. The Endowment trustees asked Few to reconsider
whether or not to attempt a four-year medical school.[11] Davison,
however, was convinced that Flexner and the Board would offer aid
in some form once they fully understood the opportunity to modernize the medical care of an entire region represented by the connection
between the medical school and The Duke Endowment. There
were, as he saw it, at least three ways open for Duke to request funds
from the Board: for a capital contribution for endowment, for
an annual grant of income, or for support of special departments of
the medical school.[12] Only the first had failed.

No hint of financial problems appeared in the initial publicity on
the medical school. The first trial balloon went up before the Durham Rotary Club on March 14, 1927. Davison was introduced to the
Durham community by University Treasurer Robert L. Flowers,
who stated on behalf of the University that Davison was to have an
absolutely free hand in planning and organizing the medical school.
The plan which Davison unfolded, based primarily on his administrative experience at The Hopkins, aimed to make Duke "better
than any other medical institution in the country." The demonstra-
ble need for physicians in the state, the absence of any preceding
school in the area, the opportunity to cooperate with the hospital
program of The Duke Endowment, the best physical equipment
money could buy, and an excellent network of roads to carry patients
from throughout the area were Duke's initial advantages. Unless his
ideas with respect to entrance requirements changed, Davison noted,
qualified students would be admitted, after two years of college
work, to a curriculum based on a quarter rather than a semester
calendar. This curriculum reform would, he suggested, enable
students to graduate in three rather than four years and reduce
the average age of graduates from 26 to 22. "We will be able to teach
students medicine here," he promised, "and know that they will go
out into the country to practice."[13]

The most important reaction to the trial balloon came from Dr.

Thurman D. Kitchin, professor of physiology at Wake Forest College School of Medicine. Kitchin charged that Davison's radical curriculum proposals constituted an attempt to enforce changes in the curriculum of the Wake Forest school. Davison assured Kitchin that this was not his intention, and reassured Few that his proposals were tentative pending their approval by the soon-to-be-recruited medical faculty.[14] This reaction to Davison's trial balloon emphasized the need, however, to explain the Duke plans fully to the state's medical profession, and to invite their cooperation, even in the planning stage, to insure its success.

As a first step in winning support from the local doctors, in April, 1927, Davison presented the plans of the new medical school to the Medical Society of the State of North Carolina. Six factors, he noted, were essential for success—the buildings, the staff, the students, the type of teaching, the service to the community, and the cooperation of the members of the profession in the state. Using slides he presented plans for the hospital and medical school buildings. The other phases, he suggested, were about to begin. Davison solicited suggestions, to be added to those made by national medical leaders, in regard to senior staff appointments. Since it was essential not only that the head of each department be a leader in his own field, but that he be a man who would have the confidence and cooperation of the physicians and surgeons of the state, Davison promised that the Medical Society members would be able to meet these men before their appointment. Aware of some resistance to the plan of employing such men on a "full time" basis, he mentioned two advantages: they would be able to devote themselves entirely to the care of patients and to the training of students and postgraduates, and they would be removed from competition with other members of the profession. All fees collected from private patients would go to the medical school and no private patients would be seen who were not referred by their own physicians. Davison also suggested that doctors practicing in the Durham area would be invited to accept part time appointments to assist in caring for patients and teaching in their areas of special competence.[15]

In discussing students, Davison shared with the Society his philosophy of medical education, developed mainly from his administrative experience at The Hopkins. Success ultimately depended, he declared, on a most careful selection from those applying for admission. Quality rather than quantity of preparation was important; two years of college, including basic science courses, was, he argued, sufficient preparation for medical school and, by lowering the age of the graduate, would permit more postgraduate internship and residency training. Statistical analyses of the performance of students at The Johns Hopkins showed that only students with no major weaknesses completed the medical course in numbers which justified the school's investment in training them: therefore, only outstanding candidates would be admitted even if this meant smaller classes and correspondingly higher tuition. Confidential recommendations from science teachers and personal interviews conducted by physicians, acting as regional representatives of the medical school, or by the dean, had proved to be the best method of selecting truly outstanding candidates. Each class at Duke would be limited to 50 students or even fewer if outstanding candidates were unavailable. Students admitted after two years who wished to take a bachelor's degree would be allowed, in their free time, to do extra work under the supervision of the medical faculty and to write a thesis to qualify for a Bachelor of Science degree.[16]

The chief advantage of rigid selectivity, Davison felt, was an increase in the liberty that could be granted the student. Medical schools had "32 months, or 128 to 132 weeks, or 4992 to 5148 hours" to impart a knowledge of medicine. With the increase in medical knowledge schools faced increasingly the problem of what to teach and what to skip. The Hopkins medical faculty decided in 1927 to meet this challenge by liberalizing its curriculum. A skeletal schedule of required courses, comprising 54 percent of the total instruction time, was devised, and students were given the choice of spreading their electives widely through the curriculum to prepare for general practice or concentrating them in one department in preparation for specialty practice. Course examinations were reduced in favor of comprehensive examinations in preclinical subjects after two years and in clinical subjects after four. The curriculum was arranged in four quarters of eight weeks each rather than trimesters of eleven weeks to provide for greater scheduling flexibility and smaller classes. With such flexibility, Davison suggested, students intending to enter practice in the South could choose a curriculum to fit the types of cases they would encounter in practice.[17]

Davison proposed to institute this Hopkins system at Duke with one major modification. He retained the quarter system but made each quarter eleven weeks long. The extra term at Duke was to be offered in the summer. By attending during the academic year and the summer a student could graduate in three years, or by attending for the academic year only could graduate in the normal four years. This proposal would not affect the curricula at Chapel Hill or Wake Forest; students taking their preclinical training at those schools over two normal academic years could be admitted to their third year at Duke either in June or September. Since those students who normally worked during the summer could be expected to earn more in the year saved by the accelerated schedule, loan funds rather than scholarships would be made available to students to be repaid after graduation.[18]

Unable to outline the teaching methods to be used pending appointment of the faculty, Davison pointed out that the connection between the medical school and the Hospital Section of The Duke Endowment would allow Duke to teach standards of medical practice which presupposed the availability of hospital facilities. The growing number of community hospitals in North Carolina, supported in part by The Duke Endowment, meant that Duke could meet its responsibility to provide doctors for rural areas without limiting its curriculum to basic instruction. In addition to providing outpatient and ward facilities "second to none" for patients within easy driving distance of Durham, Duke would also serve North Carolina by training nurses and technicians, providing consulting services, and performing laboratory procedures for the outlying community hospitals. In addition, Duke would serve the state's physicians both by providing a large medical library and by offering opportunities for postgraduate study. Doctors in the Carolinas would be able to spend days, weeks, or months at their convenience refurbishing their knowledge when necessary or learning new techniques. "The word Service," said Davison, "is to be carved into the corner stone."[19]

With his plans laid before the profession for scrutiny, Davison returned to Baltimore to wind up his affairs at The Hopkins. Few, however, urged him to continue to turn over in his mind a plan for getting more endowment for the Medical School, and Davison agreed to see G. G. Allen and Abraham Flexner about the financial resources needed to operate the new school.[20] To demonstrate its need he prepared detailed estimates of the costs of operating the medical school and hospital during the first year. He expected the hospital to serve daily an average of 100 patients who could be expected to pay one sixth of the total cost of nine dollars per patient day. Even with the Duke Endowment adding a subsidy of one dollar per patient day, the annual net cost of operating the hospital would be $244,000. Projecting a salary scale ranging from $2000 for instructors to $10,000 for full professors and $1000 for secretaries and technicians, he estimated the total budget for the medical school at $331,500, to be offset in the first year only by $30,000 in tuition fees from 76 students. The total net cost of $545,000 was higher than the corresponding figure at Vanderbilt, but less than at Rochester.[21] These were figures Flexner could understand, and he immediately promised Davison some funds for the school, although not necessarily the $250,000 per year for ten years which Davison requested. Few, horrified by the deficit, successfully petitioned the Endowment trustees to add a full fourth story to the plans for the hospital, the space to house more private rooms which would increase the annual hospital income.[22]

Davison conferred with Lewis Weed, his former chief at The Hopkins, concerning ways of securing additional funds. Davison rejected the suggestion that he should keep the six million dollars in Aluminum Company of America stock separate from University funds as a separate medical school endowment. To do so would have endangered relations with Few, to whom it was clear that "we do not have either in hand or in sight sufficient resources to develop the other departments of the University as Mr. Duke expected us to develop them and also to support the sort of medical school and hospital that the public expects of us and that all of us want to see."[23] Nor did Davison forget that the sudden failure of a railroad stock to pay dividends delayed the building of The Johns Hopkins University School of Medicine for years. He preferred to retain access to the much larger University endowment and work to attract outside funds to meet the medical school's immediate financial needs.[24]

Returning to Durham, Davison opened the first offices of the medical school on the old Trinity campus in four rooms in Bivins Hall. There the work of planning proceeded briskly as the new dean resolved a thousand and one difficulties. Plans for Few's fourth story were perfected as well as a proposal of Davison's to bend the building in the middle so that the wards would run northwest to southeast. This would provide more light and take advantage of low ground at the rear of the campus so that part of the Hospital could have seven stories.[25]

Excavation at the site increased local interest in the project, and Davison repeatedly received invitations to explain the project before local civic and professional groups.[26] With his basic plans already public, he devoted special attention to his hopes for a school of nursing. Pupil nurses, he noted, would be selected on the same basis as other Duke University women. The student nurse would have a threefold status. As a university student she would live on the women's campus, enjoy social and recreational facilities, and receive classroom instruction. As a medical intern she would gain practical experience in the care of patients. As a self-help student she would earn a part of her upkeep through service to the hospital. Davison hoped to offer, in addition to the basic nursing program leading to the diploma, a flexible curriculum which would allow the student to take a Bachelor of Science degree concurrently with or after completing the required basic course in nursing. As in the medical school itself, he noted, success would depend greatly on rigid initial selectivity.[27]

While Davison publicized his plans, the actual work of building had begun. The Endowment trustees, for legal reasons, decided that the construction work for the erection of Duke University should be done by the University rather than The Endowment, and for that purpose they chartered a new North Carolina corporation, The Duke Construction Company.[28] The company itself had a capital stock of $1000, all property, equipment, and assets used by the company being the property of Duke University.[29] As Chief Engineer of Duke University, the Endowment trustees appointed A. C. Lee, a former associate of James B. Duke's in the building of power facilities.[30] In charge of all construction, Lee was empowered to execute contracts up to $5000; Lee and the president of the company, initially University Treasurer Robert L. Flowers, could approve contracts up to $15,000; Lee and two members of the Endowment building committee initiated contracts above $15,000.[31] The total cost of buildings to be erected on the new campus was estimated at eleven million dollars. The estimated cost of the hospital and medical school buildings was $3,370,000.[32]

While the shell of the building was already on its way to completion, the University trustees resolved not to employ a faculty or incur expenses unless funds for the purpose were in hand. Bound by this resolution, Davison turned his attention to tasks which did not require additional outlays.[33] He and A. C. Lee visited hospitals throughout the eastern United States seeking ideas to improve the buildings.[34] On another tack, Davison inquired of boards of medical examiners in several states whether or not Duke students graduating under the accelerated curriculum would be eligible for state licensing examinations. Most were sympathetic to the idea of lowering the average age of medical graduates, and offered, when state law required a four-year course, at least to consider Duke graduates on their individual merits.[35] Inspection visits to Lincoln Hospital, where The Duke Endowment had made a grant for equipment purchases only on condition that Davison personally authorize all expenditures, consumed a great deal of time.[36] Also during these months Davison began to build the library for the new medical school. As no other medical schools were organizing libraries at the time, he was able to purchase bound volumes of journals at low cost. By November 3700 volumes had been ordered. The donation to the medical school of his personal library by Duke trustee J. Howell Way added extensive files of state and sectional medical journals.[37]

Forewarned by the experience of other hospitals in North Carolina, Davison also studied ways and means of improving collections from impoverished patients. In 1926 North Carolina stood forty-fourth among the states with a per capita income of $367.00 annually.[38] Many residents worked in agriculture, and therefore had small and irregular incomes. At least one-third of all patients needing hospitalization were not able to obtain it. With these facts in mind, Davison estimated that the average patient would pay only one-sixth of his hospital bills.[39]

There was a precedent in North Carolina for making collections through a prepayment plan. In 1914 Dr. T. W. Long, of Roanoke Rapids, North Carolina, had persuaded the town's six industrial employers to build and equip a hospital large enough to serve the entire community, and persuaded the employers of the plants to meet the expenses of the hospital through small, periodic contributions—which in 1928 amounted to twenty-five cents per week per employee for complete family coverage, including visits to the home, if necessary, by physicians or nurses.[40] British hospitals, with which Davison was familiar from his Oxford years, used similar plans on a community rather than a single industry basis.[41] Why not, Davison asked Rankin, organize a hospital association to provide similar coverage for residents of the Carolinas? Dues of twenty-five cents per week per family would entitle parents and children under eighteen years of age, after payment of six-months dues, to the payment of all hospital bills up to three dollars per day per person up to 21 days of care per person. Even if the average hospitalization rate of 1 person per thousand population per day were doubled, sixteen percent of collections would remain, after payment of all benefits, for operating expenses and the creation of a reserve fund. Weekly payments would be receipted by a stamp affixed to a passbook.

To insure stability of operation, the associations would be under the control of the trustees of local hospitals and admission to hospitals under the plan controlled by the hospitals. Employers would be asked to deduct dues from paychecks, prominent local citizens would be asked to serve as voluntary collectors, and a local bank would serve as treasurer of each association. Reciprocal agreement between associations might allow for coverage in hospitals in several areas of the state.[42]

Davison hoped such a plan might reduce the number of charity patients in Durham, and that county officials could be persuaded to provide funds to help cover the remainder of the charity costs.[43] He sought to enlist the support of the Durham–Orange County Medical Society, the Durham Chamber of Commerce, the Durham City Council, churches and civic clubs. As an alternative, he attempted to interest several insurance companies in offering a plan with similar features, so as to spare local communities the burden of organization.[44]

On March 14, 1929, the *Durham Morning Herald* announced that the "Durham Hospital Association" would begin operation on May 1st. The seven trustees were Dean Davison for Duke Hospital, George Watts Hill for Watts Hospital, Dr. D. S. McPherson for McPherson Hospital, Dr. Foy Roberson for Lincoln Hospital, Superintendent of Public Welfare W. E. Stanley, Mr. D. T. Carey for the Chamber of Commerce, and the Rev. J. W. Smith, representing the Durham Ministerial Association. Hospital care—not "insurance," to avoid regulation by the North Carolina insurance commissioner—was to be sold as Davison had proposed, with all payments made by the Association directly to the hospitals involved. The Security Bank and Loan Association would act as treasurer. Salvaged World War I savings stamp machines would be placed in the plants of major Durham industries to facilitate collection of dues.[45]

The announcement was premature. The Durham Hospital Association did not have sufficient capital to begin operations. Endowments and insurance companies, with no actuarial experience with this type of risk, refused to involve themselves in the Association. The insurance companies and foundations also rejected Davison's proposal that they offer a similar hospital policy, primarily because of the cost involved in enrolling individual subscribers. The question of payment charges made by individual doctors also was troublesome. Davison feared to anger the local medical profession by suggesting that they conform to a fixed fee schedule. The insurers declined, for public relations reasons, to offer a plan that covered only part of the cost of an illness or accident. The stock market crash effectively ended Davison's hopes of finding outside backing for his program. The Durham Hospital Association was stillborn.[46]

Long before the hospital care plan proved abortive, however, Davison turned his attention once again to the medical school and hospital. By August the shell of the new building was almost completed,[47] and it became necessary for him to supervise the thousands of details of interior construction so important to the efficient operation of a hospital. With A. C. Lee, he spent his days clambering over scaffoldings, doing what he could to incorporate the changes suggested by officers of other hospitals.[48] The simple addition of mechanical window openers on casement windows, for example, could save many a frustrating moment in hot or rainy weather. Proper flooring would not only reduce costs over the long run, but also reduce the noise created by the movement of patients and staff. By the end of September the cost of changes proposed by Davison and approved by the Endowment building committee had mounted to a sum estimated at more than $80,000.[49] Despite the ceiling on expenditures, there were some additions that simply had to be made while construction was in process. Attention to detail now would pay heavy dividends in the long run.

By November Davison began to organize his faculty. For months he had been soliciting suggestions, particularly from the faculties of major medical schools; now he collated these suggestions on master sheets for each department, listing for each individual his previous training, present position, the source and tenor of recommendations, and, whenever possible, the salary each person presently was receiving as well as an indication of the special research on which each was working. Duke University, he told Few, had an unparalleled opportunity to aid in the solution of five major medical care problems:

(1) the inability of most medical students to obtain adequate intern hospital training because of the average age of 26 years at which they graduate from medical school; (2) the lack of provision for intensive and extensive post graduate education for physicians who have been in practice for several years; (3) the disproportion in the distribution of doctors in the cities and rural areas; (4) the dearth of university training for nurses and (5) the need of people of moderate income for diagnostic facilities and hospital facilities within their means to pay.[50]

Securing the very best in the way of faculty to achieve these purposes would cost dearly.

With adequate funds for the operation of the medical school still not assured, Davison concluded that the School of Medicine would better meet the educational needs of North Carolina and other states if, for a period of at least five years, instead of organizing a complete medical school it would cooperate with the ten regional preclinical medical schools and their 335 students in each year, and provide training only in the clinical departments. To help the medical school and hospital meet the needs of North and South Carolina in accordance with public opinion Davison suggested the formation of an Advisory Hospital Committee composed of representative citizens of the leading cities. When in March the Rockefeller-sponsored General Education Board declined Davison's request for $250,000 annually for ten years, this scheme for cooperating with other schools seemed the only one possible.[51]

Davison was not the first Hopkins administrator to lead a new medical school, and like the heads of Ford Hospital (1919), University of Rochester Medical School (1922), and Vanderbilt University School of Medicine (1925), he recruited many of his faculty directly from among the members of the Hopkins staff. The success of this practice grew out of the uniquely high quality of scientific training given the men in residency and postresidency programs at that school. Davison relied on this procedure more completely than the heads of any of the other schools. Even those faculty chosen from positions at other institutions usually had trained or worked at The Hopkins, making Duke the most complete "colony" of The Hopkins.[52] Unable to offer large salaries, Davison found it easier to recruit able men through the existing personal relationships of a single professional group. The migration of southern medical students into northern schools for clinical studies had brought a number of southerners to The Hopkins: many of these welcomed the chance to return to make a contribution to medicine in their native region. Also, Davison recognized, a faculty whose members shared familiarity with a single pattern of educational practices and hospital working habits stood a better chance of minimizing the inevitable problems of opening a new institution.

Davison's first appointment, for Professor of Medicine, was Harold L. Amoss, a specialist in infectious diseases then Associate Professor of Medicine at The Hopkins. Davison's senior by six years, Amoss had earned the M.D. and Dr.P.H. degrees from Harvard, had worked as a chemist for several government agencies, and had spent ten years at the Rockefeller Institute for Medical Research where he was a member of the team, headed by Simon Flexner, which established the viral etiology of poliomyelitis, before joining the Hopkins faculty in 1922.[53] He had been recommended to Few by the Hopkins staff, and in a November visit to Durham favorably impressed the local physicians. Even before his appointment Davison involved him in the planning and equipping of the hospital, promising that he would have a great opportunity at Duke to carry out his own ideas.[54] Amoss agreed, suggesting that perhaps Durham would build a city infectious hospital next to the Duke Hospital, where in addition to treatment of patients, research in his specialty could be carried on.[55] After examining both the blueprints and the budget, Amoss agreed to come. At the meeting of the University trustees at which his nomination was considered, a trustee who was also a clergyman asked what church Amoss belonged to. Few, by replying immediately that Amoss's personal religion had nothing to do with his medical competence,[56] successfully eliminated the possibility of Methodist interference in medical affairs. When the appointment was announced, congratulations on the choice poured in from leading medical authorities.[57]

Immediately after Amoss's appointment was assured, Davison sent him the list of candidates for positions in the department of surgery, noting three names which he felt should be considered most seriously for the professorship.[58] His policy was to include each full professor in the process of selecting other full professors. He and Amoss agreed to recommend Julian Deryl Hart for the professorship. A native of Georgia and a bachelor, Hart held B.A. and A.M. degrees from Emory University, the M.D. from Johns Hopkins, and was then completing his eighth year of residency in surgery. Especially competent in mathematics, Hart would be useful, beyond his specialty, in administrative consideration of financial matters. They also selected, as professor of pathology, Wiley D. Forbus, a Washington and Lee graduate who, after two years of private school teaching in Washington, entered The Johns Hopkins and received his M.D. in 1923. An associate in pathology at The Hopkins, his work as visiting pathologist of the Baltimore city hospitals and consulting pathologist of the Frederick City Hospital would be valuable in setting up consulting laboratory services at Duke for the community hospitals of the Carolinas.[59]

The appointment of a chief nurse proved most sensitive. At the November, 1928, meeting of the Association of American Medical Colleges Davison had asked for a vote on whether the administration of the medical school and hospital should be separate, with the Dean in charge of the medical school and the Medical Superintendent in charge of the hospital, or whether the Dean should be responsible for both, with a business manager in charge of the financial and other details of both. Seventy-eight of the eighty deans at the meeting advised Davison to accept administrative responsibility for both in the interests of harmony and efficiency, despite the increase in personal work load.[60]

This advice also applied to the selection of a nursing supervisor. A chief nurse with years of experience in making administrative decisions could save the dean a great deal of time, but an older woman, very positive in her likes and dislikes, also could cause irritation within a newly formed staff of comparatively young doctors. As early as November Davison had sounded out for the position Miss Bessie Baker, whom he had known while in Europe in 1917.[61] An experienced Hopkins-trained nursing administrator, Miss Baker was a former Assistant Superintendent of Nurses at The Hopkins and currently Superintendent of Nurses at Miller Hospital in St. Paul, Minnesota. As with the other candidates for appointment as department heads, the dean shared his plans with her and asked for her suggestions. Impressed with the brisk professionalism of her replies, he selected her for the position after conferences with Amoss, Hart, and Forbus where it was agreed that the department heads would be able to appoint their own supervising nurses for their departments.[62]

With the appointment of these department heads Davison's personal work load trebled. Most complex was the task of equipping the medical school and hospital. The inventory lists of the medical schools of The Hopkins, Rochester, and Vanderbilt were compared and combined to form master lists for each department. For the rooms and laboratories of Duke which these lists did not fit, lists were made from suggestions of friends at The Hopkins.[63] In consultation with the department heads, each room was assigned to either Medicine, Surgery, Pediatrics, Administration, or Dietetics, and a set of cards was prepared showing the equipment to be installed in each room, attempting whenever possible to define standard units of equipment for similar rooms, and the cards sent to the appropriate department head for further suggestions. Once the lists were complete, Davison had to consolidate the information on the cards to be able to place orders through A. C. Lee for each item in the desired quantity.[64] Where suggestions involved changes in the building itself, as in the installation of electricity, pipes, vents, major appliances, or new doors, Davison had to act as liaison between the department heads and the engineers, while purchases of equipment had to be timed to meet construction schedules. Each detail had to be recorded and repeatedly checked by Davison personally.[65] One whole week was devoted to making sure that every door was of the right size and opened in the proper direction. As there were 1447 doors in the Medical School and Hospital, he told Amoss, it was a bewildering task, but he recalled that there was nothing more annoying than to try to push a 3′6″ bed through a 3′ door, as he occasionally had to do in the Harriet Lane.[66]

After the appointment of "Miss Bessie," Davison considered it wise not to make any announcements of additions to the staff until later, since there had been some discussion among the profession about the concentration of Hopkins-trained staff. The selection process continued unabated, however, Davison and Amoss being in agreement to take the best suited man regardless of his origin.[67] Each department head was given the responsibility for final selection of his staff, often selecting from the lists of candidates provided by Davison, and the department heads as a group chose new men of rank comparable to their own.[68] Candidates for lesser positions were chosen from Davison's lists, and since many were at The Hopkins, Amoss, Hart, and Forbus were able to act as on-the-ground recruiters. William A. Perlzweig, chemist to the medical clinic at The Hopkins, was chosen Professor of Biochemistry. Edwin P. Alyea, appointed instructor in urology, and Watt Weems Eagle, instructor in otolaryngology, were quickly recruited from among the instructors on the Hopkins staff. From the Hopkins laboratories came technician Mary Poston. From the Hopkins hospital came Mildred M. Sherwood, Chief Pediatric Nurse, and Marian F. Batchelder, Chief Operating Room Nurse.[69] Mrs. Elsie Martin, professor of dietetics, previously was administrative dietician at the Lakeside Hospital in Cleveland. Former Hopkins resident Alfred R. Shands, Jr., left his position as attending orthopedic surgeon at four Washington, D.C. hospitals to become instructor in orthopedics, and Baylor-trained Robert J. Reeves, instructor in Roentgenology, was chosen from the Columbia faculty.[70] Davison personally chose Marcellus E. Winston, Business Manager of the Park View Hospital in Rocky Mount, North Carolina, for the position of Superintendent of Duke Hospital, and brought him to Durham to help with the equipment purchases.[71]

Only slightly less complex than selecting the faculty was the stocking of books for the medical library. Davison and a niece of Endowment trustee William R. Perkins, Miss Judith Farrar, who had been appointed medical librarian, and her mother, Mrs. Mildred Farrar, compiled cards showing the holdings of the Hopkins, Rochester, Vanderbilt, and Boston medical libraries and collected these on a master list. Appointees and friends in each specialty were asked to grade each item on the list as "necessary," "desirable," or "useless," and the recommendations on each item were compared. Bids for those items considered necessary or desirable were solicited from fifty-seven medical book dealers throughout the world. It was decided that any price under three dollars per volume was generally acceptable, and that more expensive purchases would be studied individually. At the same time a list of journals for current subscription was compiled and initial subscription orders placed.[72]

At the same time, Davison reopened negotiations with the Rockefeller Foundation. Public expectations and the desire of Duke University and Duke Endowment officials to be faithful to the intentions of James B. Duke would not allow development of a purely clinical medical school until all possibilities for funding the full four-year school were exhausted. Although the dream of additional millions in endowment or income was gone, Davison still hoped that, with buildings already available for housing the first and second years of the medical school, the Foundation might grant sufficient income to help maintain them for the first five years, when hospital and medical school receipts would be lowest. Estimating the annual operating cost of preclinical instruction at $116,650, Davison asked for five annual grants of $100,000, $80,000, $60,000, $40,000 and $20,000, respectively for the years 1930 through 1934, so that preclinical instruction could commence from the opening of the school in 1930. Since the application did not fall within the present policies of the Foundation, it was referred once again to the General Education Board. Abraham Flexner and Trevor Arnett, President of the Board, were sympathetic to the request. The Board, however, wished to be thoroughly convinced that the University was assured of adequate funds available to maintain the hospital, clinical instruction in the medical school, and all other departments of the University on the highest level, so that it could operate without further recourse to the General Education Board or without finding itself in an embarrassing situation later.[73]

Davison and Few planned their strategy carefully. Citing the need of a four-year medical school in the region and the expectations of the state that he operate such a school, Few presented fully Duke's financial position and let the Board judge as to its adequacy, pointing out that in the fiscal years 1927–1929 additions to endowment and loan funds would total $2,313,000. To help answer the question of who controlled the medical school, he published a short pamphlet, *The Duke Endowment and Duke University,* in which he presented the Endowment trustees as, in a vital sense, University trustees charged to see that the University remained true to the purposes for which it was founded. Quoting at length from the indenture which created The Duke Endowment, he noted that funds to the University could be shut off only for fiscal irresponsibility, and personally promised that "while we could profitably use more funds than we have, we are going to cut our garments to the cloth."[74] Davison noted that low labor costs in Durham, provision by the University of centrally supplied utilities and housing for nurses on the women's campus, the charity payments and funds for equipment and library contributed by The Duke Endowment, and the Angier B. Duke Loan Fund, which would allow the medical school to receive full tuition from every student, would keep costs lower than at comparable institutions like Vanderbilt and Rochester.[75] Discussion continued throughout the summer; Board President Arnett, fully converted, requested an additional twenty-five copies of Few's pamphlet for distribution to Rockefeller officials.[76] At their November meeting the Board approved Davison's proposal. "We need the money," Few wrote Toms, "but the implications are even more valuable to us now than the money."[77] "It is," he told the University trustees, "even more significant as an indication that American philanthropy and the American public will not withhold gifts from Duke University because one man has made it a very great gift."[78]

With funds in hand for preclinical instruction, Davison expanded the recruiting process. The salaries Duke could offer were not high: professors started at from $5000 to $7500 annually, some with promised increases to $10,000 by 1934; associate professors drew $3500 to $4500; assistant professors received from $3000 to $3500; instructors up to $2500.[79] Along with modest salaries, new faculty members could expect to have a great deal of work in setting up new facilities and programs. There were, however, the freedom to develop one's own ideas and to advance rapidly in academic rank. Each candidate was considered not only on the basis of his scientific qualifications but also in terms of his potential loyalty to the University. Men who gave the impression of using a Duke position only as a stepping-stone were not invited to the campus and no position was ever offered to anyone who did not first indicate that he would accept it if an offer were made.

There were two additional department heads, Hopkins-trained Francis H. Swett of Vanderbilt as professor of anatomy and George S. Eadie of Hopkins as professor of physiology.[80] Also from The Hopkins came assistant professor of medicine Oscar C. E. Hansen-Prüss, instructors Roger D. Baker in anatomy and Frederick Bernheim in physiology, surgical residents Clarence E. Gardner, Jr., and Robert R. Jones, pathology resident Earle B. Craven, and anesthesiologist Mary Muller.[81] The residents, over Miss Baker's objections, would live with their families in the empty rooms of the fourth floor of the hospital.

Some of the Hopkins-trained appointees brought with them ideas and experience gained elsewhere. Bacteriologist David T. Smith, director of the research laboratories at the New York State Hospital at Ray Brook, became Duke's professor in charge of bacteriology and associate professor of medicine. His wife, Susan Gower Smith, joined Perlzweig in the Department of Biochemistry. Duncan C. Heatherington accompanied Swett from Vanderbilt to take charge of histology and neuroanatomy. Wilmer Institute chemist Haywood M. Taylor also joined Perlzweig's biochemistry department as an assistant professor. Bayard F. Carter, Professor of Obstetrics and Gynecology at the University of Virginia, agreed to head up that department beginning in 1931. Until his arrival Durham obstetrician Robert A. Ross would serve as acting head. Some had no Hopkins experience. Carter brought with him from Virginia endocrinologist Edwin C. Hamblen. From New York's Bellevue Hospital, gastroenterologist Julian M. Ruffin joined the Department of Medicine as assistant professor. Christopher Johnston, instructor in the department of medicine, Ernest McCutcheon, instructor in dentistry, and medical resident Elbert L. Persons had no previous connection with The Johns Hopkins.[82]

Three of North Carolina's most prominent medical personalities also joined the new faculty. Winston-Salem neurologist Frederic Moir Hanes became associate professor of medicine. Watson S. Rankin accepted an appointment as a visiting lecturer in preventive medicine and public health, and William deBerniere MacNider, Dean of the University of North Carolina Medical School, contributed his special talent to the organization of the courses in pharmacology. Also as he had planned, Davison extended invitations to Durham physicians to accept part-time, unsalaried appointments in the out-patient department. To local physicians not offered such appointments he extended private patient admitting privileges. In part these were public relations gestures aimed at lessening resistance to the idea of a permanent faculty paid "full-time" salaries. He hoped, however, to be able to use the best qualified among these men to relieve permanent staff of their responsibilities in the out-patient department for one academic quarter in each year.[83]

As in the other departments of the University, a tight budget had dictated a young faculty. "Too large a proportion of them," Few wrote to Perkins, "are young men who have not yet won their spurs."[84] Davison, however, found confidence in the fact that Osler was 39, Halsted, 37, Welch, 34, and Kelly, 31, when first appointed by Daniel Coit Gilman to lead the original Hopkins faculty.[85] Now, in a similarly new situation, the Hopkins's latest young progeny were eager to try their hands.

Applications from students had to be processed even more rapidly than appointments of faculty. The Council on Medical Education and Hospitals of the American Medical Association, acting on the recommendation of its chairman, Ray L. Wilbur, gave Duke a Class A rating in 1929, even before buildings and faculty were complete, on Davison's assurance that the appropriate standards would be met.

Announcements of the school's opening, rating, and entrance requirements were placed in college newspapers.[86] By January of 1930, 500 applications had been mailed out, and another 1000 were being printed. The original admissions policy called for all but obviously unworthy candidates to be screened by a committee of Davison, Amoss, and Forbus. With Davison and the applications in Durham and Amoss and Forbus still in Baltimore, however, this seemed to Davison too cumbersome a procedure involving too much correspondence. He therefore took responsibility for admitting or declining candidates, following the practices he helped to establish at The Hopkins.[87]

The publicity announcements circulated by the university also sought students for the schools of dietetics and nursing, schools which Davison planned should provide personnel immediately for Duke and gradually for the hospitals cooperating with The Duke Endowment. The school of dietetics offered a one-year course of class instruction and practical experience leading to a Certificate of Graduate Dietitian. The basic nursing course, three years of eleven months each, awarded a Diploma of Graduate Nurse. Davison had planned to accept the work of the pupil nurses in the hospital in lieu of any tuition fee since all other North Carolina hospitals paid nurses a bonus and he feared that the charging of a tuition might be too startling an innovation. Miss Baker, however, felt that a tuition fee would attract "a higher type student." She had her way, and tuition of $100 was charged. By vote of the University faculty, the School of Nursing was authorized to grant the Bachelor of Science degree to women who completed two years of acceptable college work before or after, but not during, the three-year nursing curriculum.[88]

The problems Davison confronted in organizing the building of the medical school and hospital made him vividly aware of the potential need for trained hospital administrators in the community hospitals supported by The Duke Endowment. After conferring with Watson S. Rankin and Michael M. Davis, a medical economist who was about to publish a book entitled *Hospital Administration, A Career,* Davison decided to offer to graduates in Business Administration a two-year course which combined orientation in the health and hospital field and an application of administrative principles

to the operaton of hospitals, teaching primarily through work experience at Duke which would relieve Davison of some administrative legwork.[89]

As the medical buildings neared completion, they became a sight-
seeing attraction for the entire community. As many as 3000 to
4000 people viewed the construction on a single Sunday, some gaz-
ing wonderingly at the size of the buildings and others peering
curiously at the details of the symbols of hope and faith and the seals
of the American College of Physicians, American College of Surgeons, and university medical school carved above the entrances.[90]
Davison fed the wondering and the curious with a steady stream of
press releases describing the buildings and their functions. The first
floor of the medical school would house administrative offices, the
medical library, the pharmacology department, and a student health
unit under the direction of Dr. Joseph Speed. Biochemistry and
physiology classrooms and laboratories would occupy the second
floor, the bacteriology and pathology departments and autopsy facilities the third, anatomy and histology the fourth, with pens for experimental animals on the fifth and in the loft. The close proximity
of the medical school and hospital would allow students to move
easily between the classrooms, the laboratories, and the wards.[91]

Onlookers found the hospital even more fascinating, since it promised to affect their lives more directly. Covering four acres of ground
with 20 acres of floor space with a total capacity of 416 beds and 50
bassinets for newborn infants, it was located away from noise and
urban conditions yet within easy access of highways in all directions.
Its first floor housed the out-patient services, emergency room, administrative offices, male medical wards, dining rooms, and the
amphitheater. Male and female private rooms and 16-bed wards,
divided into white and colored sections, were on the second floor.
On the third floor were the male surgical wards and physicians'
offices, connected by a corridor with the pathology laboratories in
the medical school. On the fourth floor were obstetrical, gynecologi-
cal and female surgical wards and the operating rooms. Initially,
however, only the second-floor rooms would be used for patients—at
least until a mounting census demanded the opening of additional
space.[92] Ward beds would cost $3.00 per day, semiprivate $4.00, and
private $5.00 to $9.00. Additional charges would be added for special

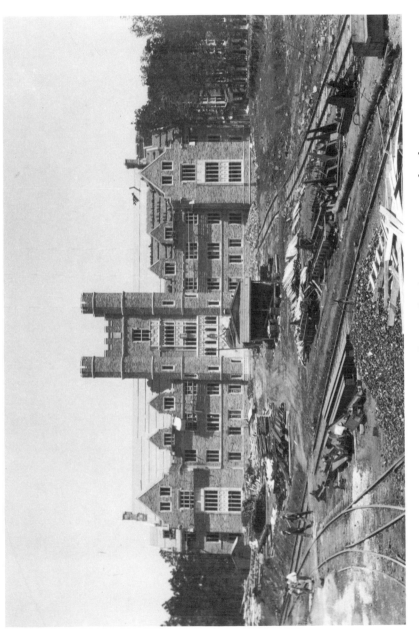

Medical School construction, 1928—the towers are completed

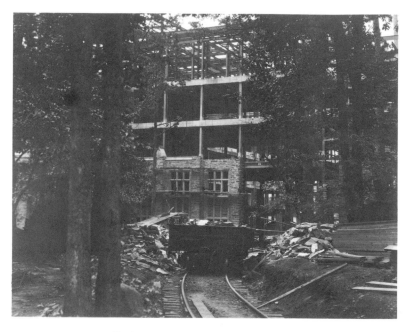

Duke Hospital construction, 1928

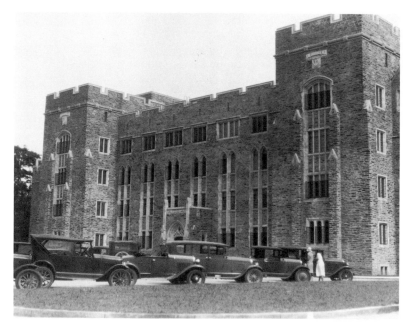

Duke Hospital completed, 1930

services, such as laboratory tests, x-rays, or operating room. An advance payment covering estimated hospital charges was to be required of all patients, and a letter of introduction from one's personal physician was recommended. Physicians were encouraged to accompany their patients to the hospital. Patients seeking reduced rates or charity care were to be required to submit certification of their inability to pay from county welfare officials. The outpatient clinic, open daily for whites from 1:30 to 3:00 P.M. and for colored from 3:00 to 5:00 P.M., would charge a basic rate of $2.00 per visit with special procedures extra. Davison estimated the total annual cost of running the hospital at $280,000 annually.[93]

The formal opening of the hospital was scheduled for July first, but delays caused by failure of equipment to arrive forced Davison to postpone the opening to Sunday, July 20, 1930. The day dawned hot and humid. Practically everybody suffered, the *Durham Morning Herald* reported, especially during the afternoon when the temperature reached its high of 95 degrees. From nine o'clock in the morning until five o'clock in the afternoon a crowd finally estimated at between 15,000 and 25,000 persons examined every nook and corner of the mammoth structure.[94] Davison lost six pounds and ruined a white linen suit showing visitors through the building and repairing overloaded elevators.[95]

The hospital was opened to patients on July 21, and had in the first weeks of its opening many more patients than even Dr. Davison had hoped or provided for.[96] Twelve patients were admitted to the hospital and five were treated in the out-patient clinics on the first day, the first among them A. C. Lee, the chief engineer of the Duke Construction Company.[97] By September 1589 patients had registered at Duke, of whom 254 were admitted to the hospital.[98] In the first six weeks after opening, the surgical staff performed a total of 121 operations, 77 major and 44 minor, an average of three per day.[99] This heavy work load severely taxed facilities still not fully equipped or organized and forced postponement of plans for a formal dedication of the medical school.

Davison's original intention of placing all of the medical faculty on a full-time salaried basis, as at The Hopkins, had been modified because of the low budget available for salaries. On the advice of Harvey Cushing and Henry A. Christian of the Harvard Medical

School, a "geographic" full-time plan was adopted for members of the clinical staff. Under this policy members of the medical faculty were free to conduct a private practice, and to charge fees, at Duke Hospital, but were to devote their full time to work done at the Duke Hospital and Medical School.[100] At first the rewards of this practice were not large. Only 23 percent of the patients registered were under the private care either of one of the Duke faculty or of a personal physician.[101] Only half were able to pay the full charges for their hospital care, and approximately one-fifth of all patients were unable to pay anything.[102] "We get," Few told Perkins, "a good many echoes of hard times."[103]

On September 1, the Executive Committee of the Faculty of the School of Medicine and Hospital, composed of the heads of the departments of the medical school, met officially for the first time. This committee was the key link in the chain of committees through which Davison controlled the medical school and hospital, giving its advice and consent on matters of policy and appointments, delegating subcommittees to provide for decentralized handling of administrative problems such as curriculum and visiting lecturers, and acting on all appeals or protests from faculty, staff, or students. Davison served both as secretary and adjutant to this committee, translating its decisions from his minutes into hospital and medical school policy. For the first few months this committee spent most of its time establishing the standard procedures necessary for efficient hospital operations, largely based upon the Hopkins patterns, which had developed almost out of habit since the hospital opened in July. Procedures for distribution of drugs and of experimental animals, admission of patients, requisition of supplies, and performance of autopsies, as well as working schedules for the staff and hours for the out-patient clinic quickly were given formal approval.

The other committees performed more specialized functions. An Administrative Council of the Hospital, consisting of the President and Treasurer of Duke University and the Dean of the Medical School, interpreted the decisions of the Executive Committee and the financial needs of the Medical School and Hospital to the Executive Committee of the Duke University Trustees, which finally approved or disapproved the budget and all appointments. Allocation of funds within the limits of the budget was left to Davison alone. On financial matters he dealt with department heads individually rather than through the Executive Committee. With money in short supply and only Davison able to compare the importance of departmental proposals in light of the total funds available, this arrangement gave him complete personal control of medical affairs at Duke. A sub-committee of three of the University trustees, the Advisory Hospital Committee, periodically evaluated the purposes, scope, and quality of work done at the hospital and recommended extensions of operations and improvements in service to the trustees. Later an administrative committee for the hospital, consisting of the deans of the schools of medicine and nursing, hospital administrator, professor of dietetics, admitting officer, and chairmen of the clinical departments was established to manage matters pertaining to patient care, with the hospital superintendent acting as adjutant. A nursing committee chaired by the Dean of the School of Nursing performed a similar function in that area. Finally, all members of the medical school and hospital staff who held University appointments, including residents and interns, constituted a Faculty Committee through which "matters of routine" were handled and decisions of the Executive Committee discussed. All of these committees and councils met once a month.[104]

Only Davison sat on all the committees, in order to coordinate the objectives and methods of each department within the priorities he had established for the entire University medical division and which the senior staff had accepted prior to their appointments. The immediate need of North Carolina for physicians, the work load in the hospital, and the lack of funds designated specifically for support of research dictated that the first priority of the medical school and hospital must be its teaching programs. Second priority would go to maintaining quality service to patients, the third priority to the training of technicians from among the local populace, and way down in fourth priority came research designed to increase understanding of the diseases and other problems faced in the hospital.[105]

Thirty first-year and 18 third-year students, selected from some 3000 applicants, arrived on October second to begin their studies.[106] With initial enrollment far below the capacity of 70 students per class, the faculty resolved to develop teaching methods based upon individual relationships with students. The apprentice system of teaching used at the University of Wisconsin Medical School was investigated as a potential model for training the general practitioners needed in the Carolinas by assigning students as externs in physician's offices to gain experience with the problems of the physician in competitive practice and the importance of environmental factors in understanding and treating patients.[107] Most students found the work hard and the standards high. At the end of two quarters 13 first-year students received "strong warnings" stating that unless their work improved markedly they might be forced to withdraw from the school. Another 14 first-year and six third-year students received "mild warnings" indicating that their performance level was low in one or more courses and that improvement was advisable. Even so, the executive committee allowed the students to choose between proctored examinations and an honor system. In April the honor system was instituted.[108]

Despite the interest and excitement aroused by the problems of teaching, the operation of the hospital continued to be the primary occupation of most of the staff. In the first months of 1931 an average of 640 patients registered each month at the hospital or out-patient clinics; of these, an average of 250 were admitted.[109] The number of nurses required to care for the patients rose from 22 in August, 1930, to 72 in March, 1931. With each nurse receiving a base pay of $80.00 plus a room and board allowance of $25.00 per month this increase placed additional strain on an already tight operating budget. Except for the hospital kitchen, no other department increased its staff more than 20 percent during this period, but overtime work became increasingly common in the administrative offices.[110] Senior staff, in addition to their responsibilities to students and patients, also faced the problems of training local people to serve as technicians in the laboratories and of observing the everyday work of their departments, reducing each operation to an efficient routine, and presenting the routine to the Executive Committee to be approved as hospital policy. In addition, good personal and public relations required senior staff members to meet the people of Durham, the University community, Duke Endowment officials, and area physicians. "We spent much time," Dr. Forbus later recalled, "cultivating the acquaintances and good will of groups we would be dependent on."[111]

Community good will helped, but financial problems remained most pressing. The hospital simply could not give charity treatment to all who applied. Plans for expansion throughout the University, as well as the necessity of supporting both the Law and Medical Schools during their first years, when receipts from tuition would be low, dictated that the University could not use its funds for the hospital ward care of charity patients other than those with conditions of medical or surgical teaching interest. Patients whose incomes were less than $15.00 per week were asked to apply, through their family physicians, for examinations in the out-patient clinics. The clinics educated the public about proper medical care, treated part-pay and free patients whenever possible without using hospital bed space, and screened patients for teaching purposes. Three patients were examined in the clinics for every one admitted to the hospital, yet the deficit continued to grow. In April, Few told G. G. Allen of the Endowment trustees that the Medical School and Hospital sorely needed additional funds.[112] The large deficit was, in part at least, a measure of the hospital's success. A patient load far greater than expected was now being served efficiently.

With the initial period of organization finally completed, plans were laid to hold the long-delayed formal dedication of the Medical School and Hospital. At Davison's invitation the State Medical Society was to hold its annual three-day meeting in Durham. April 20, the first day of the convention, was given over entirely to the dedication exercises. The morning and evening sessions were opened to the general public.[113]

The morning exercises were dominated by the memory of James B. Duke. George G. Allen, in presenting the buildings to the University on behalf of The Duke Endowment, recalled that Mr. Duke expected to be looking down upon his work one thousand years hence. Dr. Thurman D. Kitchin, President of Wake Forest College, who had once expressed fear that the Duke curriculum would harm the state's two-year schools, now pledged the complete sympathy and cooperation of North Carolina's medical profession to the end that Mr. Duke's dream might be fulfilled. Dr. David Linn Edsall, Dean of the Harvard Medical School, pointed out the immediate benefits of the Duke facilities by describing "the birth of a new medicine" dominated by the exact knowledge gathered in scientific laboratories and applied to the eradication of disease. In the evening Dr. William H. Welch, "silver haired and impressive," challenged the new school to pursue prevention of disease in the South through the scientific study of medicine with the same zeal which characterized his contemporaries on the original young Hopkins faculty.[114]

Davison's former chief at The Hopkins, Dr. Lewis H. Weed, speaking at the afternoon session to an audience limited to invited guests, best summed up what the combination of the Duke benefactions and the Hopkins-led revolution in medicine could mean. Duke University, he noted, established its medical school at a time when medical educators, partially in recognition of the rapidly increasing scope of knowledge in each clinical and preclinical department of medicine, generally were opposed to standardization of the medical curriculum and were content to grant each school latitude of individual development. The increase in medical knowledge and its accompanying equipment, coupled with the rising cost of "free" care of hospital patients, promised to increase substantially the cost of medical education. Only the future could judge the worth of Davison's conviction that better physicians would be produced at less overall cost in a program that decreased the number of years spent in study and increased the number spent in hospital or laboratory internship. For the present the excellent research facilities and the spirit of self-education at Duke were enough in themselves to justify the experiment. "If anything augurs well for the success of this great undertaking in medical education," Weed concluded, "it is, in my opinion, the research spirit of the originating faculty and its willingness to start on an educational experiment as expressed in its curriculum, not following blindly the tested arrangements of other schools, but sailing out, in part at least, on the unknown sea of educational procedure."[115]

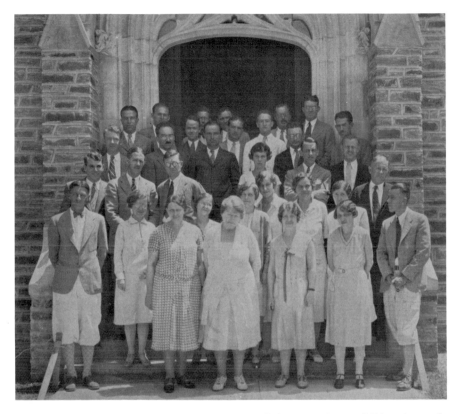

Original Staff, Duke University Schools of Medicine, Nursing and Dietetics, and Duke Hospital, July 19, 1930 (two days before the opening).

First row (left to right) : Dr. Bellows, Mrs. Martin, Mrs. Sykes, Miss Baker, Miss Patrick, Miss Laxton, Dr. Swett

Second row (left to right) : Dr. Eagle, Dr. Alyea, Dr. Forbus, Miss Batcheldor, Miss Floyd, Miss Nelson, Mrs, Lawlor, Miss Muller, Dr. Amoss

Third row (left to right) : Mr. Smith, Dr. Perlzweig, Dr. Oates, Miss Robinson, Dr. Hansen, Dr. Johnston

Last two rows (left to right) : Dr. Gardner, Dr. Ziv, Dr. Jones, Mr. Reese, Dr. Magill, Dr. Craven, Mr. Ward, Dr. Davison, Dr. Taylor, Dr. Hart, Dr. Reeves

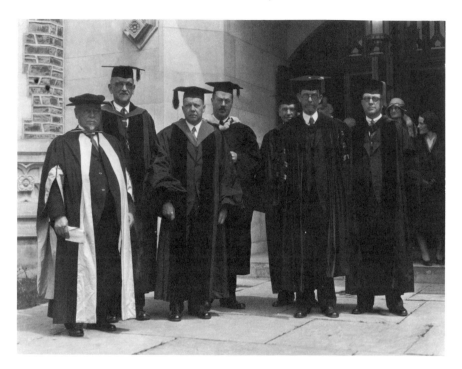

Dedication, Duke University Medical School, April 20, 1931. *Left to right:* Dr. William Welch, Johns Hopkins University; Dean David Linn Edsall, Harvard University Medical School; Director Lewis Hill Weed, Johns Hopkins School of Medicine; Dean Wilburt C. Davison, Duke University School of Medicine; Dean Elbert Russell, Divinity School, Duke University; President William Preston Few, Duke University; President Thurman D. Kitchin, Wake Forest College; Dr. Watson Smith Rankin, Director of Division of Hospitals of The Duke Endowment, not shown

Part Two: The Regional Medical Center, 1931–1941

Chapter 5: Experiments in Cooperation: Financing Medicine During the Depression Decade

The most pressing problem to emerge during the first year of operation of the Duke University School of Medicine and Hospital was the inability of patients to pay the cost of their care. This reflected a national condition, with origins prior to World War I, which national medical authorities were only beginning to study. Wilburt Cornell Davison, together with members of the Medical School staff and Watson S. Rankin, director of the Hospital Section of the Duke Endowment, designed and largely implemented a system of financing of medical care which provided access to scientific medicine for all persons, whatever their economic status. This system not only anticipated national trends in medical financing and accounting, but also promised to give the Duke University School of Medicine and Hospital financial control of their own future.

Between 1914 and 1927 rates charged by American hospitals rose almost 100 percent,[1] as a consequence largely of wartime inflation and the need for increased capital investment in new medical technology, such as laboratory equipment and x-ray machines. Physicians' fees rose not only with the cost of living and the prestige of the profession but also with the increased investment, in time and money, necessary to gain and sustain a medical education.[2] As the costs of medical care rose, persons with low incomes received less and less care, and suffered proportionately. Patients of moderate means, unable to pay comfortably the full cost of unexpected or prolonged illness, tended to choose medical charity rather than financial tragedy, and collection of bills became a major problem for hospitals and doctors alike. Many younger physicians located in cities, where the newest technology was available to them in large hospitals, creating an imbalance in the availability of medical care between town and country. By 1927 the gap between the cost of medical care and the purchasing power of most of the American people created a loud public outcry.[3]

The depression did not create, but did appreciably deepen, the crisis over the cost of medical care by increasing the number of persons who could not pay their bills. In 1930 the net income of private physicians dropped 20 percent from the level prevailing in 1929. Americans spent a larger percentage of their income for medical care in 1931 than in 1929, but in dollars they spent less by more than 13 percent.[4]* An estimated 38 of every 100 white Americans, concentrated particularly among the poorer classes and in the South, received no medical care at all. Among Negroes over half received no treatment.[5] For nine of every ten families, even before the depression, the burden of unexpected major medical expense was too heavy to bear.[6] Patients seeking free care placed a heavy burden on all hospitals, but particularly on voluntary private hospitals, whose income from endowments and contributions decreased during the depression by two-thirds while the charity load increased almost fourfold.[7] An annual expenditure of $82 per family per year would provide adequate medical care on the average for the American people, exclusive of dentistry; nine of every ten families, before the depression, could afford this amount.[8]

In 1927 The Committee on the Costs of Medical Care, a private group which included doctors, public health officials, economists, and representatives of the general public, was organized to study, over a five-year period, the economics of American medicine and to propose means for the delivery of adequate, scientific medical services to all the American people at a cost within their means to pay.[9] The ultimate solution suggested by the Committee was to provide nearly every city of over 15,000 persons with a "community medical center" which would include a general hospital, pharmacy, outpatient department, laboratory service, and well-stocked library; in short, all facilities and services necessary for the practice of scientific medicine. The Committee recommended smaller hospitals or medical sub-stations for rural areas, staffed by groups of local physicians but supervised by the specialists at one of the community medical centers, where all difficult cases would be treated. The plan

* Americans spent $2,937,000,000 for medical care in 1929, as compared to $2,549,000,000 in 1931, but in 1931 this represented 4.27 percent of their income as compared to 3.34 percent in 1929. These figures reflect the necessary character of major medical expenses in an elastic market: physicians fees dropped 15 percent while hospitalization expenses dropped less than 2 percent.

promised to reduce the general overhead of medicine by providing many services at one location; it would help eliminate waste by providing a central control over expenditures for medical service in an entire area; it would also make it possible to offer a quality of care, both to ambulatory and hospital patients, which would reduce the hidden costs of illness, such as loss of time from work, by reducing the average length of incapacitation and increasing the prospects for complete recoveries.[10]* The Committee recommended the use of tax funds to cover the cost of care for those unable to pay and insurance to help middle income families make the high cost of sudden illness a budgetable item.

All of the economic problems facing American medicine nationally affected the operation of the Duke Hospital. In the fiscal year 1930–31 Duke University paid as a subsidy to the Hospital, over and above funds from all other sources, more than $260,000, or almost as much as Davison's early estimate of the *entire* cost of operation for the first year.[11] The average daily patient census was almost 150 and rising, but only one of every four white patients, and one of every 25 Negro patients, who made up one-sixth of Duke's patient load, was able to pay the full cost of treatment.[12] The Medical School did not yet have a full student body, so receipts from tuition were still below normal. Senior staff members were not receiving the salary increases promised at the time of their appointments. University income was reduced by the depression: among the endowment investments which stopped paying dividends was the Aluminum Company of America stock which secured the Medical School's income.

Davison and Rankin foresaw most of the problems, although not their total effect. During the planning stages they had more control over the means of delivery of medical care than over any other single factor affecting total medical costs. They therefore had included in the plans for the Duke Hospital the first major out-patient clinics in North Carolina. Patients of limited means who were not

* A minority of the Committee opposed group practice as destructive of the personal relations basic to the art of medicine and insurance as inviting lay interference in medical practice. Initially, a majority of the nation's doctors seemed to agree with the minority report. *Medical Care for the American People,* p. 151ff.; Richard H. Shryock, *The Development of Modern Medicine,* pp. 419–20.

acutely ill were referred to the appropriate specialty clinic by a social service worker or admissions officer. At the clinic a medical student, intern, or resident secured from the patient a complete medical history and performed a physical examination, urine and blood analyses and a chest x-ray. Once the study was completed, the student conferred with a senior staff member as to what additional diagnostic procedures were necessary, what course of treatment was to be recommended, and whether the patient required hospitalization. The patient then was referred back to his personal physician, to whom a letter was sent summarizing the personal history, and diagnostic procedures and the recommended course of treatment. The cost to the patient was minimal; collections during the first decade averaged less than fifty cents per visit. The low cost was possible because large numbers of patients could be accommodated in small amounts of space and time by a limited number of salaried people.[13]

The completeness of the examinations offered to patients and the value to the physicians of the area of diagnostic assistance in difficult cases quickly made the out-patient clinics the most important single means of enlarging the hospital's patronage (see Figure 1). Hospital admissions officers frequently were embarrassed by well-to-do patients seeking care at low cost in the belief, based partly on their reputation for giving complete examinations, that the clinics, like The Mayo Clinic, were open to everyone.[14] Fourth-year medical students working in these clinics taught their patients basic health procedures and gained experience in diagnosis and treatment of patients under conditions which closely simulated general practice.[15] New mothers, for example, were taught to prepare lactic acid evaporated milk for their children to guard against harmful bacteria common in the well water and unrefrigerated whole milk used in rural areas.[16] The clinics served the hospital as a device for screening patients for admission to the wards, insuring that bed space went first to the most acute cases and identifying patients with problems useful for teaching and research purposes. The clinics soon outgrew the space and schedule allotted for them in the original plans (see chapter 4 above). Only by scheduling clinics in the mornings as well as the afternoons, constantly rearranging the original space, and converting an additional basement wing into

Figure 1. Duke University Hospital, growth by services to patients

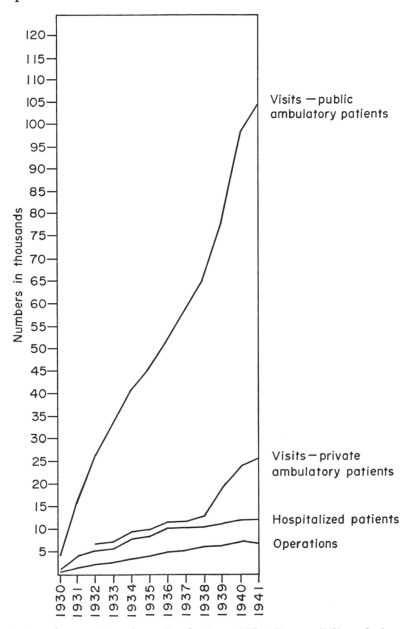

Visits — public ambulatory patients

Visits — private ambulatory patients

Hospitalized patients

Operations

Note—figure taken from Deryl Hart, "The Responsibility of the Medical Profession to Medical Education," *Annals of Surgery* 145 (May, 1957) : 615, and included by permission of the editors.

examining rooms were the thousands of patients per month accommodated.[17]

The rapid growth in the patient load of the public dispensary, the time required for care of ward patients, an eleven month teaching year, and individual and group research projects combined to severely limit the private practice from which the clinical staff members had expected to derive the major portion of their income. During the depression even private patients often paid belatedly, or not at all, many choosing not to return to Duke rather than pay what they owed. And the doctors, pressed for time, were not adept at raising the percentage of charges collected. Without the breadth of clinical experience which comes from long years of practice, the Duke doctors often found it necessary to consult with each other in the diagnosis of difficult cases, complicating the problem of distributing equitably the limited receipts from private patients. There was need to expand the clinical staff beyond the limit of one physician per subspecialty imposed by the University budget so that staff members could take vacations and set aside their patient responsibilities long enough to do the study necessary for effective teaching. To compete for good teachers with institutions in large cities where a private practice might seem more certain to materialize, Duke would have to guarantee new staff members an adequate initial income.[18]

As a solution to these problems Dr. J. Deryl Hart, Professor of Surgery, proposed the creation of a voluntary cooperative group practice to include the members of the clinical staff. Such an organization, he suggested, would insure the best possible diagnosis in complicated cases through wide consultation and exhaustive diagnostic laboratory procedures wherever necessary. To reach this goal, Hart recognized, a schedule of fees would have to be established for all medical services and consultations. The fees of necessity would be low; similar ideas had failed elsewhere because consulting physicians insisted on high fees in every case, leaving little income for the primary physician and reducing proportionately his readiness to call on colleagues for consultation. Yet the fees could not be so low as to undercut the charges of the local medical profession. As an example, Hart offered to set his top consultation fee for patients seen under such a group practice arrangement at ten dollars. Where the patient could pay only part of the charges made for his treatment, Hart noted, the doctors and hospital must agree to accept the same percentage of the amount collected as they would if the whole bill were paid.[19]

Supported by Dr. David T. Smith, acting head of the Department of Medicine, and Dean Davison, Hart presented his ideas to the full clinical staff. Some were reluctant to limit their private practice in this fashion and, despite assurances that the individual physician alone would decide which of his private patients would be handled under the group arrangement, exactly half of the clinical staff opposed the proposals. Those opposed, however, were fairly evenly divided among the medical departments, and two days of intensive lobbying by Davison, Hart, and Smith produced favorable majorities in each.[20] On September 15, 1931, the clinical staff organized the Private Diagnostic Clinic. The name reflected the fact that Duke University, although it housed the Clinic, was not engaged in the private practice of medicine.[21]

Since no provision for a clinic for private ambulatory patients had been included in the original building plans, the P.D.C., as it was called, opened in improvised temporary space. Patients coming to the Clinic for the first time were given complete work-ups, including the taking of physical examinations, medical and financial histories, and basic laboratory tests, before being referred to the appropriate senior staff member. This doctor called for whatever additional consultations and laboratory procedures he found necessary and recommended the course of treatment. All financial arrangements, however, were handled by a business office under the direction of W. F. Franck, a former real estate dealer and insurance agent who knew from his past experience many of the central North Carolina families with sufficient resources to pay for their care. Collections were handled on a purely business basis, quite apart from the close personal relationship between patient and physician. In this situation patients paid more and complained less often. Free from work-up and collection responsibilities, the doctor spent only half as much time with each private patient, a situation which together with the larger percentage of charges collected raised his income even after deductions for clinic overhead and allowed him more time for his other responsibilities.[22]

Once the Clinic was established, the department heads manipulated the financial mechanism to solve a variety of problems. The first problem centered around income protection. Under the original agreement within the Department of Medicine, for example, each doctor received the entire professional fee paid by his patient less a percentage deduction toward the overhead of the Clinic. Originally 22.5 percent, this deduction was gradually reduced as the Clinic grew to 11 percent. Under this arrangement, however, if a man stopped working his income stopped. The doctors were reluctant to take time off for study or vacation. To combat this, Dr. Frederic M. Hanes, who in 1933 had succeeded Harold L. Amoss as Chairman of the Department of Medicine, proposed the creation of a Department of Internal Medicine fund.

Under this plan Hanes and the other members of the department pooled all fees collected from private patients. Hanes, an independently wealthy man, took no percentage of the pool for himself. Each of the other members of the department received every month a percentage of the pool, after the deductions for overhead, equal to the percentage of collections he contributed during the previous year. Each man was allowed one month each year for study and one for vacation. At Smith's suggestion a "50 percent up or down clause" was added to the basic arrangement. If in one year one doctor's contribution to the pool was ten percent higher than what he received from the pool, the following year his receipts from the pool were raised by five percent. If his contributions decreased ten percent, the next year his earnings from the pool were reduced by five percent. This device rewarded industry and at the same time cushioned the impact of illness or other misfortune on a man's earnings. No man's dollar income was reduced during the decade, however, because of the continuing increase in the total business of the department.[23]

Once every faculty member was assured an adequate and regular income, the financial mechanism was altered to increase professional opportunities and to improve general working conditions. By 1936 the total income of the Department of Medicine had grown sufficiently for Hanes to propose the establishment of a fluid research fund for the Department of Medicine. Since part of the income from private patients accrued from the name, prestige and facilities of the Duke Hospital and School of Medicine, he argued, a reasonable part of such earnings should be allocated to a medical research fund for the use and betterment of the whole department. The members of the department agreed that a research tax of five to ten percent should be levied on the net incomes derived from private practice of the more prosperous members of the senior staff. They gave Hanes authority to raise or lower the tax on an individual's income based on his total net income from private practice, his teaching load, and his contribution to research during the preceding year. The higher a man's research productivity, the lower his research tax. Collections, made each month by the Business Manager of the P.D.C. and deposited in a separate account, in the first three months amounted to $3400.[24]

Mrs. Anna H. Hanes, the mother of the professor of medicine, donated $5000 to establish the Anna H. Hanes Research Fund early in 1937, and Hanes himself immediately donated an additional $7000. The research tax paid by the members of the Department of Medicine, additional gifts from the Hanes family, contributions from Duke University, and money given by foundations and private industry to support research by members of the department swelled the Hanes Fund in the months that followed. The Hanes Fund provided salaries for technicians and secretaries, as well as instruments and supplies needed for teaching and research, which were beyond the limited University budget. Gradually a reserve was accumulated which was used to match, and thus in fact to attract, new grants from outside sources.[25]

This willingness of the clinical staff voluntarily to invest in the future of the institution found its most important expression in an increase of staff. In all departments the P.D.C. arrangements allowed Duke to guarantee a competitive minimum income to new faculty members. The Department of Surgery, for example, as originally organized included three assistant professors in orthopedics, urology, and otolaryngology, who derived their private income from the practice of those specialties, and Hart, who alone carried general, thoracic, plastic, and neurosurgery, the "core group," as he called them. When in 1932 Dr. Clarence E. Gardner, Jr., joined the staff in general surgery, Hart divided the total income from "core group" practice with him on a percentage basis. Each time a new man joined the group another redistribution was made.[26] Similar arrangements prevailed in the other departments.

The income of new men varied considerably according to specialty and patient load, but in the Department of Medicine it was expected that they would earn at least $7500 annually, of which the University paid only one third.[27] The University placed no limit on the amount its clinical staff could earn from private practice, an arrangement which kept the incentive to practice constant and intense. Once established, faculty members in their turn were expected to allow a part of their private earnings to be used, through the percentage distribution agreement within the department, toward the development of another young teacher. By so doing they not only helped to improve their own departments but also released a larger proportion of University funds for use in attracting competent instructors for the preclinical departments, whose members did not share in the P.D.C. arrangements and were paid full-time salaries by the University.[28]

During the first five years all of the clinical departments used the same collections machinery under a single business manager. Each department made its own charges, the business office collected them, subtracted its costs, and passed the funds on to the departments, and the members of each department determined how their funds were spent. Methods for accomplishing the same purpose varied considerably from department to department. The Department of Surgery, for example, financed its additional technicians, secretaries, and equipment not from a general tax but from a pool of fees either given by patients to whom the surgeons extended courtesy service or collected from charity patients, too poor to pay their overall hospital bill, who could pay something directly to the doctor.[29]

By 1937, however, the growth of the total private practice and the dissimilarity of the needs of the departments of medicine and surgery led to an administrative separation of the P.D.C. into Medical and Surgical Divisions. The surgeons, who derived most of their income from treatment rather than diagnosis, wished to keep diagnostic fees, laboratory overhead and office expenses low. Doctors on the medical side, who saw larger numbers of patients and depended upon diagnostic service for their income, had proportionately greater need for these facilities. To meet these divergent goals the P.D.C. divided into two financially autonomous divisions, each able to al-

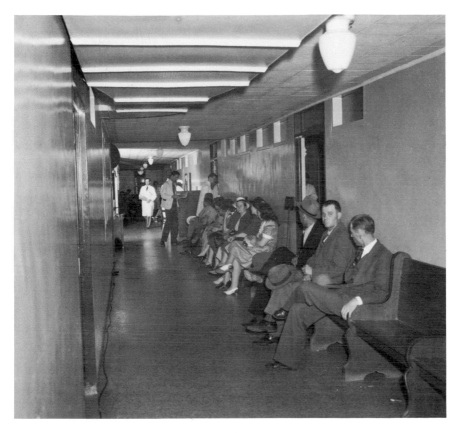

Medical Clinic, May, 1941

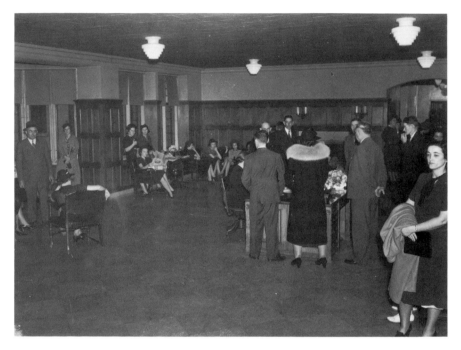

Duke Hospital lobby, November, 1938

locate its resources to meet its particular needs and each with its own business manager and office. The patient, however, dealt only with one P.D.C., even if he saw doctors in both divisions. In such cases the schedule of fees for consultations and the agreement to divide income on a *pro rata* basis were kept intact, and the distribution of receipts was handled by the business manager. So well had the value of separating collections from care established itself that the doctors turned over to the business managers for collection the accounts not only of patients seen by more than one staff member but of their individual private patients as well.[30]

As the number of doctors engaged in private practice increased as a result of the success of the Private Diagnostic Clinic, and as the demand for charity care continued to soar, the number of private beds available to each man who was supposed to earn most of his living from private practice dropped to approximately three.[31] By 1939 the mounting number of private ambulatory patients also made necessary more private examining rooms than could be crowded into the temporary space which housed the P.D.C. To meet these needs, the University and The Duke Endowment agreed to add a wing to the Hospital which would provide more private and semiprivate beds and also one floor of offices and examining rooms for each of the two divisions of the Clinic.[32]

The University could not supply the examining area rent free and proposed that the Clinic pay an annual rental of $17,500 for this space. Some of the doctors objected that this violated the original agreement between the University and the medical staff wherein the University agreed to furnish space for the private practice of the staff as part of their compensation for teaching.[33] The medical staff proposed instead that in addition to assuming all the expenses of operating the Clinic they would, in lieu of rent, put into a building and development fund for the Medical School and Hospital a percentage of the income from private practice (initially four percent of the gross) to yield a sum greater in amount than the proposed annual rental. By this arrangement the University benefitted by an increased return on its investment and the medical staff was assured of more beds and increasing facilities in the Medical School and Hospital.[34] Since the general prestige of the University helped to attract private patients and since the University neither limited nor inquired into the income derived from private practice, most doctors paid this small price gladly.

The clinics could not, however, relieve the pressure on the Hospital budget caused by patients requiring hospitalization who could not pay their bills. Two-thirds of the hospital care given at Duke in 1931 was entirely free, and the demand for such care was increasing.[35] Many persons misunderstood the charitable purpose of The Duke Endowment and assumed that it supported the Duke University School of Medicine and Hospital. Patients who received free care told their friends and relatives about it, with the result that Hospital admitting officers faced more frequent demands for free care with each turnover of patients. Prodded by large deficits, both Hospital and University officials recalled James B. Duke's philosophy that complete charity prostituted the character of the people while wise aid could and should assist them in obtaining services superior to what they themselves could afford. Clearly, the percentage of persons paying part of their bills had to be raised if the Duke Hospital was to remain solvent.[36]

The original billing policy of Duke Hospital was to charge patients a daily rate for room and board plus an additional sum for each service rendered by the hospital, a system of billing which became common in American hospitals between 1910 and 1930 as a convenient means of passing on rising wholesale costs.[37] In 1932 Davison sent F. Vernon Altvater, one of the first two students in Duke's Hospital Administration Internship Program, to study methods of financial administration, bookkeeping, and collection at several major midwestern medical centers[38] to prepare him to succeed Marcellus E. Winston as Superintendent of the Duke Hospital. Upon his return Altvater analyzed over 700 patient accounts and discovered that the average patient remained in the hospital for 12.8 days, was charged an average rate of $5.20 per day, but actually paid only an average of $1.77 per day for his care. This low collection rate had developed, Altvater reasoned, because hospital costs could not be estimated in advance on a room and board plus extras basis. And once having left the hospital, the patient, his income reduced by the depression, found it too easy to demand charity. Just before he succeeded Marcellus E. Winston as Superintendent of Duke Hospital, Altvater presented Davison with a detailed plan for a "flat rate" or "inclusive" billing system. Duke Hospital, he suggested, should charge a flat rate for each day of care which included most extras. Such a plan would allow hospital admitting officers to calculate charges at the time of admission and enforce payment in advance.[39]

The plan helped the patient as well as the hospital. From his sample survey Altvater found that there was little difference between departments in the average per diem charges made to patients. A single rate for each class of room, private, semiprivate, or ward, therefore could be applied to patients on each service. The private surgical patient who under the room and board plus extras plan paid $149.50 for his operation, one x-ray, and 19 days of care would pay under the inclusive plan $128.25. A ward medical patient presenting medium diagnostic difficulties would pay no more than $49.20 for 14 days of care which otherwise would cost $67.50. After considering the patient's ability to pay, the admitting officer might admit him to a ward for as little as a dollar a day. The Hospital's financial position would be improved, since it would be able to collect in advance an average bill of $2.62 per day. A collection rate of 70 percent of charges would enable the Hospital to raise sufficient funds, above fixed income, to cover operating costs. In this financial position the Hospital could afford to expand its census and serve more people more rapidly, even if this meant an increase in the gross dollar value of charity care rendered. The flat rates could be adjusted upward or downward to correspond to general economic conditions, and lower flat rates could be offered on those services needing to attract more patients. Two factors, Altvater noted, were essential for the plan's success. Admissions at less than minimum rates or without payment of charges for at least 15 days in advance could not be made. He predicted also that a large amount of initial publicity would be necessary to explain the merits of the plan to avoid alienating a public not yet accustomed to meeting its responsibilities for medical care on a pay-as-you-go basis.[40]

When Davison and Altvater shared their proposal with Dr. Rankin of The Duke Endowment he was immediately sympathetic. The plan possessed two virtues even beyond the administrative and financial benefits to Duke Hospital. The flat rate system tended to reduce the uneven burden of the costs of treatment by spreading the costs of most special procedures across the entire patient population, a feature fully in accord with the recommendations of the Committee on the Costs of Medical Care. More important, it presented an opportunity to offer all the people of North Carolina a chance to participate, through their elected representatives and influential groups, in the statewide medical services offered by the Duke Medical School and Hospital and The Duke Endowment. Why not, Rankin suggested, request each county government to appropriate a fixed sum of money to be spent, at the rate of one dollar per patient day, for the care of charity patients treated at Duke who were unable to be hospitalized in their home county. Simply presenting figures on the amount of charity care given at Duke Hospital to county commissioners would help to develop intelligent popular understanding of the costs of medical care and the work of the University and The Endowment. And if the figures were presented, not for coercion, but as an invitation to participate in a large beneficent program, by sharing the cost of treatment with the Hospital and The Endowment, that understanding could be translated into both good will and financial support.[41]

The plan was not without potential dangers. Other hospitals might object that Duke was attempting to lure their patients away by offering less than competitive rates. More important, it was questionable whether truly indigent patients, especially in rural areas, could raise even minimal advance payments from relatives, friends, or charitable institutions. Professor of Biochemistry William A. Perlzweig cautioned that if Duke adopted the plan and in consequence large numbers of patients were turned away, popular condemnation of the institution would be boundless and not counteracted by any degree of publicity, paid or otherwise.[42] Painfully aware that during the first months of 1933 prices for farm crops were as low as they had ever been, Perlzweig argued that some patients would have to be treated entirely free.[43]

For four months Dean Davison and his new superintendent, Altvater, worked to perfect their proposal. Invitations to county governments to assist Duke in offering charity care would coincide with publication of a report showing that in 1932 the counties contributed only one-half of one percent of the cost of charity treatment and with a public announcement of the flat rate schedule. Other hospitals were almost certain to object to the new rates or to publication of the amount of charity care being done by Duke for patients from their areas. In Durham Davison expected opposition from Watts and Lincoln Hospitals, both private institutions, which were incurring operating deficits despite limited aid from state and local governments. Dr. Rankin and the Duke Endowment trustees approved of the plan, however, particularly for its educational value.[44]

In April Altvater put the new system into effect. Private patients were charged $6.00 to $9.00 per day, depending on the type of room occupied. Persons such as clerical workers, with limited but steady incomes, and all patients covered by insurance were charged $3.50 for ward beds and $4.50 for semiprivate cubicles. Both of these groups were expected to pay professional fees in addition, but the Duke staff members were encouraged to set their fees for the second group in accord with their ability to pay. The Hospital charged ward patients at least two dollars daily.

Both Altvater and Perlzweig proved to be partly right and partly wrong. When the word first spread that "it costs two dollars at Duke" out-patient clinic patronage fell briefly.[45] There were persons who simply could not pay or raise two dollars per day for their care, and Altvater in these cases had to bend his standard. By making clear to patients that Duke Hospital adjusted its charges according to the patient's ability to pay, however, he succeeded in establishing the standard on a more flexible basis than he first envisioned, and patient volume quickly returned to normal. Public acceptance encouraged Davison to promote a wider patronage. He asked Rankin about the advisability of publishing a small advertisement of Duke Hospital rates in all the North Carolina papers. Aware that advertisements could be a boomerang,[46] he nonetheless decided that the opportunity for Duke Hospital to render much larger service to North Carolinians, made possible by and insuring the success of the flat rate system, should not be allowed to pass.[47]

The notice as it finally appeared announced both the flat rates and the willingness of the Duke Hospital to enter into cooperative arrangements for meeting the cost of medical care for the poor. One day of hospital care cost in excess of $4.00. If a patient's family, friends, church, lodge or county welfare department paid $2.00, in advance, then Duke Hospital would cooperate and pay the other half. Patients were asked to write, or to have their physicians do so, before traveling to the Hospital.[48]

Almost immediately both Rankin and Davison began to receive the inquiries they had feared from physicians and officials of other hospitals questioning the propriety of this action.[49] Rankin put his personal prestige on the line in defense of Davison's action. His counter-attack was ingenious. First he pointed out that no solicitation of patients was made nor were comparisons drawn between Duke and other hospitals. Then he argued that with the charity load at Duke Hospital approaching 90 percent, it was necessary to impress the public and public officials with the limits of the charity Duke could offer. Finally he clinched his case by putting the critics on the defensive: the new requirements for payments in advance of admission made it imperative to give the public the same knowledge of the admitting procedures that physicians had received earlier through professional journals such as *Southern Medicine and Surgery* and the *Virginia Medical Monthly*. It was only fair, he concluded, for patients not referred by physicians to receive adequate warning against traveling long distances to Duke only to be turned away when unprepared to pay.[50]

Many physicians, however, remained irritated. The North Carolina State Board of Medical Examiners notified Davison that, in their opinion, an advertising campaign was a mistaken policy.[51] In an editorial, *Southern Medicine and Surgery* spoke of "the publishing of these rates of charge in the public print as an exceedingly regrettable incident, one which promises of little good." No hospital in the Carolinas, the journal noted, could afford to match the Duke rates.[52] This was true because Duke, as a teaching hospital, was already routinely performing a large number of diagnostic procedures per patient, whereas at other hospitals the increase in such procedures that flat rates would bring threatened to raise costs alarmingly. Moreover, the number of procedures requested by an outside staff under flat rates could not be controlled by the hospital where the members of the staff were not on a "full-time" basis.

To reduce the widespread criticism among physicians in the area, Davison contemplated requesting the State Medical Society to appoint a "Duke Hospital Guidance Committee" to investigate complaints and explain Duke's problems to the public. He also considered reinstituting an earlier policy of telephoning the physician of every charity patient who applied for admission in order to learn whether the physician recommended the patient's admission.[53] It was painfully evident that both physicians and hospitals were acutely sensitive to financial competition because of the depression.[54] On the other hand, in the absence of adequate credit-reporting facilities in rural North Carolina, some patients who paid full rates at home were able to gain charity admission at Duke despite the requirement of letters from physicians, welfare officers, or ministers, credit reports, and sworn statements of financial condition.[55] This practice Duke Hospital had to stop, but with its reputation for riches, Duke could not afford to appear overly competitive.

Despite the agonized outcry from physicians and hospitals, the publicity devoted to the cooperative plan began to achieve its goals. In 1932, only 13 of 86 counties sending patients to Duke Hospital assisted them financially, but in 1933, 68 of 91 counties recognized some degree of financial obligation towards the care of their indigent.[56] The money contributed by the counties was slightly more than five percent of the cost of their care.[57]

The cooperative plan prescribed that only emergency charity patients should be admitted to Duke Hospital from Durham and counties which did not recognize their obligation to pay half of charity patient costs. One-third of the charity work done by Duke Hospital in 1932 was for the people of Durham, at a cost in excess of $90,000,[58] yet neither city nor county contributed toward the cost of free care for its citizens. University funds could not be stretched to cover so large an expense for so long, nor could the University afford to allow Durham to accept the services of the Duke Hospital as charity if it were to be successful in asking other municipal governments to pay part of the costs of care for their indigent patients.

The financial problems of Durham County were severe. At Watts Hospital the charity work load increased from 22 percent in 1929 to 65 percent in 1932. A survey by the Durham Health Department revealed that four of every ten Durham residents could not even afford to pay for home care by a physician, a statistic corroborated by reports from Durham doctors that half their fees were not collectable. The valuation of taxable property in Durham County was expected to drop approximately $200 millions, and a tax increase of twenty cents per $100 valuation was necessary just to maintain the salaries of school teachers at existing levels. Both the city and the county were expected to reduce their appropriations for support of Watts Hospital. Some of the County Commissioners felt that Duke should receive its fair share of public funds for local charity patients. Because the number of charity patients at Duke was so large, however, prospects for aid, either from the city or the county, were poor.[59]

Supporters of Watts Hospital initially opposed any appropriation for Duke. Watts, they argued, was Durham's hospital, and as long as it had beds available and was in financial need all city and county funds should go there. George Watts Hill, a trustee of Watts Hospital, warned the County Commissioners that the hospital donated by his grandfather might fail as a private institution if adequate support for charity care were not provided. Duke, he argued, commanded large outside support, admitted charity patients to be studied by medical students, and did not allow all local physicians to practice there.[60] Duke's case, on the other hand, was a strong one. Duke Hospital, warned the County Commissioners that the hospital donated County, and The Duke Endowment paid another 28 percent. Certainly bearing so large a share of the burdens entitled Duke to a proportionate share of what public funds were available.[61] In 1934, therefore, when George Watts Hill asked the city and county governments for an appropriation of one dollar per patient day of charity care given Durham residents, Davison considered it only fair that Duke should be given the same support as Watts and Lincoln, in proportion to the amount of charity work done,[62] and made a similar request for funds.

Effective consummation of the cooperative plan ultimately depended on finding a satisfactory definition of the working relationships between Duke Hospital and Durham, and among the Durham hospitals. Four of every five Durham charity patients treated at Duke were brought there by physicians. The Duke medical staff may have assumed that they did so because of the superior staff and facilities to be found there. But when the *Durham Morning Herald*, in support of the cooperative plan, commented that "Duke Hospital can offer certain services Watts Hospital cannot," a Watts Hospital partisan, understandably piqued, retorted that the Watts staff was "not so highly specialized but probably more humane and charitable."[63] The city council, caught in the middle, first appropriated $7500 for treatment of charity cases at Duke on a dollar a day basis, then reconsidered and eliminated the appropriation from the budget. After further backing and filling, the council once again reinstated the appropriation with the provision that Watts and Lincoln be designated as Durham's charity hospitals, leaving only "emergency" cases to Duke.

Controversy then arose over the definition of "emergency." George Watts Hill contended that Duke should be restricted to accident cases, but Davison felt that acute medical cases and cases which Duke was uniquely equipped to treat should be included.[64] The Durham–Orange Medical Society, invited by the city council to help arrive at a workable solution, resolved not to enter into "controversy with newspapers or city officials in regard to the classification or hospitalization of local charity patients, or in regard to the relative ability of local hospitals to care for charity patients."[65] The controversy over the definition of "emergency" concerned not only current funds, but also future appropriations. Some city councilmen felt that the designation of Duke for charity hospitalization purposes might open the door to other types of financial requests from Duke Hospital. Others feared that unworthy residents might take advantage of the provision and claim free care improperly.

When Durham County appropriated $5000 for charity hospitalization at Duke without the "emergency case" limitation, opposition to the city's restriction mounted. Watts Hospital was drawing city funds for charity care, but in the absence of a working definition, Duke was not, despite the fact that in the first 90 days after the appropriation authorizing payments to Duke, 1600 days of charity care were given at Duke to city residents. Private negotiations between Davison and city officials, from which the press was excluded, dragged on for six months.[66] Finally they found an acceptable formula. Funds not to exceed $4000 were appropriated to Duke Hospital for the fiscal year 1934–35 for the treatment of full charity accident or emergency cases. The council resolved that such cases were to be "strictly interpreted" and personally approved by the

Superintendent of Duke Hospital.[67] This formula allowed Duke to collect funds due for care extended since the initial appropriation passed, brought Durham into line in principle with the goals of the cooperative plan, and by setting a limit on the expenditure, quieted those councilmen who feared assuming any financial responsibilities at Duke. In actual practice, of course, the upper limit on the appropriation meant that Durham city and county would not pay the two dollar daily rate because of the large number of patients seeking care.

Public awareness that Duke Hospital charged according to the patient's ability to pay rather than according to the actual cost of treatment helped to establish in the public mind the concept that every individual should contribute at least in some measure to the cost of his medical care. Between 1932 and 1938 the percentage of patients unable to pay the full cost of their care remained constant at 87 percent, but the percentage of costs paid by these patients rose from 24 to 57 percent. This improvement resulted in part from the general business recovery and in part from the shorter average length of a single hospital stay[68] (see appendix 1). Under the flat rate plan, over 90 percent of charges made, to both private and charity patients, were collected.[69] Under the cooperative plan, 71 of 99 counties assisted their indigent patients at Duke in 1938, together paying six percent of the total cost of charity care of the Hospital.[70] In Durham, city and county fixed appropriations for charity care were sufficient to cover only half of the basic rate of two dollars daily because of the large number of patients requiring treatment.[71] The generally improved collection rate, however, combined with the reduction in the average length of stay, allowed Duke Hospital to treat more and more patients using the same fixed endowment.

The Private Diagnostic Clinics offered Duke patients who could afford to meet their medical bills ready access to specialists in group practice and the most modern medical facilities. The cooperative plan, through the out-patient clinics, provided charity patients with access to the same services at little or no cost to themselves. To the person of limited means, loath to accept charity yet unable to meet the high cost of sudden hospitalization, insurance offered a means of making medical care a budgetable item. Davison's first experiment with insurance, the Durham Hospital Association, had failed before the Duke Hospital opened for want of operating capital. His second, a proposed Duke University Medical Guild, was a group coverage plan for University employees which called for pooling the medical bills of the community and paying them, through payroll deductions, on the basis of equal shares per family enrolled.[72] This plan failed because some members of the Duke faculty, fearing unanticipated costs under the scheme, persisted in looking for "jokers," and the experiment languished from too much tinkering.[73]

The publication of the reports of the Committee on the Cost of Medical Care during the years 1928 to 1933 stimulated new interest in health insurance plans. Graham L. Davis, an assistant to Rankin on the Duke Endowment staff, for several years had promoted the concept of hospitalization insurance among North Carolina doctors and hospital officials.[74] In 1933, however, two plans derived from Davison's original Durham Hospital Association idea entered the field. In Durham Mr. B. S. Smith, encouraged by philanthropist George Watts Hill, attempted to organize a group payment plan for hospitalization but failed to win the approval of the Durham–Orange Medical Society. In Raleigh, Marcellus E. Winston of Rex Hospital, formerly Superintendent of Duke Hospital, helped to interest Mr. Dwight Snyder, a group insurance salesman, in organizing the Hospital Care Association, Incorporated, which was chartered by the State Legislature in August, 1933. The Hospital Care Association was the fourth nonprofit hospital plan to be incorporated in the whole United States, and, according to Davison, the first successful plan to envision statewide operations.[75]

Duke and Watts Hospitals immediately agreed to extend credit in the amount of $1000 over eighteen months to the new company, and George Watts Hill provided its first cash operating fund by endorsing a note for $250. Each hospital was allowed to name one member of the Association's board of directors. Drawing on the earlier contacts made by Hill and Davison, Hospital Care then enrolled some 3000 members, or 95 percent of its total membership, including the faculty and staff of Duke University, through its Durham office. In November, the Durham branch became the organization's headquarters.

The Association's contracts for hospital care provided 19 days of care per year to start with, increasing two days per year for each year a contract remained in force to a maximum of 30 days. The contracts were sold by commissioned salesmen, primarily to employee groups but also to individual persons and families. Initially, to attract as many members as possible, no restrictions for existing pathological or obstetrical conditions were placed upon members, as the organizers felt that a broader base of enrollment would spread the risk over a sufficiently large and healthy population. The contract covered room, board, general nursing care, routine laboratory work, operating room or delivery room charges, x-rays, and dressing and medicines administered in the hospital, but excluded physicians' fees, special prescriptions and laboratory work, and private nurse's charges. At private room rates this cost a man and his wife $18.00 per year. The Hospital Care Association paid hospitals $6.00 per day for a $5.00 private room and ancillary services.[76]

Almost immediately, however, the Association began to lose money. The actuarial experience of the company far exceeded predictions, especially at Duke. Of the first 701 certificate holders, 264 were in the Duke group. Probably because they were more aware than the public generally concerning the benefits of hospitalization, they used Duke Hospital far more than was anticipated. The managers of the Association complained that the hospitals kept the patients longer than necessary, and appealed to physicians to help reduce the average length of stay, and thus reduce the Association's losses.[77] The 1934 operating deficit of over ten thousand dollars indicated, however, that a more thorough reorganization was necessary.[78]

In February, 1935, the Duke and Watts Hospitals each furnished the Hospital Care Association with $6000 for guarantee capital which was immediately used to buy out the original stockholders and pay off the company's debts. New by-laws provided that the Association could assume special obligations in favor of the two hospitals in return for cash or credit advanced. Through this arrangement the hospitals would absorb future operating deficits of Care by advancing additional credit in the form of extensions on payments due the hospitals. Under the new by-laws Duke and Watts Hospitals named five of seven directors of the Hospital Care Association, including all of the Executive Committee.[79]

With the aid of F. V. Altvater, Duke Hospital superintendent, the Association installed new recording and accounting procedures to allow statistical study of each group contract. Nine of fifteen employees, including the original manager, Dwight Snyder, were released and a new manager, Mr. Donald E. Deichmann, was hired. To make the Association self-supporting without raising rates, certificates issued to new subscribers excluded dependents from coverage during the first two days of any illness. A married couple would pay $21.60 for coverage at private room rates or $14.00 for ward rates, with an additional premium of $2.40 annually for each child under fourteen and higher premiums for older dependents. Having enrolled almost 20,000 members from the professional and white-collar classes by the autumn of 1936, the Association then attempted to fulfill its original purpose and enroll the working classes. A new low cost certificate was offered which provided up to 25 days of care in the ward for an annual premium of six dollars. Most white "charity" patients, it was thought, could meet an average premium of less than two cents per day. A separate certificate offering more limited benefits was offered Negroes at less cost. A registration fee of one dollar for each certificate was charged, which helped to reduce the administrative costs of doing business. The Association reserved the right to cancel any contract at the end of any period of premium payment, thus providing a mechanism for eliminating uninsurable risks.[80]

In 1936, after a year of operation under the new scheme, the Association again operated at a deficit of just over ten thousand dollars, but where in 1934, with 4734 members, this represented a loss of $4.30 per member per year, in 1936, with 22,500 members, the average loss was $0.66. "The only trouble with this damn business" said its president, B. W. Roberts, "is that it is dying of improvement."[81]

As the reorganization proceeded, new competition emerged. The continuing discussions among members of the State Medical Society and the North Carolina Hospital Association concerning the feasibility of a statewide hospital care prepayment plan led both groups to form study committees, which joined under the chairmanship of Dr. I. H. Manning, Dean of the School of Medicine of the University of North Carolina. Manning and Graham L. Davis traveled to England to study hospitalization plans.[82] Their reports moved the joint committees to apply to The Duke Endowment for financial assistance for a new statewide prepayment plan for bringing hospital care within the means particularly of workers and others unable to meet the full costs of unexpected illness.[83]

Rankin and Davison both were anxious to have as many North Carolinians as possible covered by hospitalization insurance. Since the Hospital Care Association lacked the funds for immediate statewide expansion and because many doctors in the state, preferring that the medical profession as a whole control health insurance, labeled the Hospital Care Association "socialized medicine," the application was approved by The Duke Endowment. A new corporation, The Hospital Saving Association, opened headquarters in Chapel Hill.[84] Competition between the two plans quickly took on the intensity of the not unrelated rivalry between Duke University and the University of North Carolina. Although the new plan quickly surpassed the Hospital Care Association in total membership, both continued to lose money. The influential *Textile Bulletin*, while accepting hospital insurance as good in principle, actually advised North Carolina textile plants editorially to postpone purchasing group hospitalization plans for their employees until the associations were financially sound and were regulated by the Insurance Commissioner of North Carolina.[85]

Officials in nearby states watched the competition to see if hospitalization insurance offered on a statewide basis could succeed. The American Hospital Association, which accredited such plans by allowing them the use of the Blue Cross symbol in advertising, also watched, concerned that the competition neither reduce the total number of persons enrolled nor adversely affect the development of similar ventures in other states. The A.H.A. forced both Hospital Care and Hospital Saving to submit to outside audit, and then to consider plans for a merger. The two associations agreed to form a control board composed of three members of each association and a permanent executive controller, with power to direct competition, regulate salaries, hire and fire employees, oversee financial matters, set rates, and approve or disapprove expenditures while maintaining the separate identity of the two associations. Their bitter rivalry, however, would not allow either to assume the debts of the other and allow completion of the merger. The talks dragged on month after month, but by 1940 both associations began to realize substantial earnings. The Hospital Care Association's first real profits enabled it to begin repaying Duke and Watts Hospitals the $34,500 each had advanced for underwriting the Association. Once this happened both sides lost all interest in merger.[86] Not until 1968 would the two plans finally unite.

The five experiments in the financing of medical care made at Duke during the depression decade made a crucial contribution to the success of the institution, even though only one of them produced substantial revenue. Many of the staff contributed to the individual experiments, but the pattern as a whole was Davison's creation, the product of his continuing effort as dean to keep the Medical School and Hospital solvent. His goals were to reduce, by voluntary cooperation wherever possible, the costs of medical care to the patient and to increase the benefits of practicing medicine at Duke to the physician. The out-patient clinics were an experiment only in the sense that they were new to the region. The clinics made it possible to accommodate much of the overwhelming demand for charity care at minimal cost to the patients. By reducing to a minimum the staff, space, and time required for accurate diagnoses, a wide variety of clinical problems were screened for teaching purposes and the physicians of the area gained the benefit of the best hospital facilities available for difficult diagnoses while retaining the initiative in the treatment of their patients. Altvater's flat rate scheme distributed the costs of hospitalization more evenly over the patient population, and by increasing the percentage of charges collected, correspondingly increased the number of patients who could be treated at Duke on a partial cost basis. The cooperative plan enlisted the aid of families, friends, community organizations and, most importantly, local governments in making quality medical care available to the indigent, while the Hospital Care Association helped to make North Carolina one of the first states where Blue Cross insurance was everywhere available. And each time an individual citizen, physician, or government official participated in one of these experiments he also looked to Duke as the region's leading medical center.

Of all the experiments, the most important was the Private Diagnostic Clinic. By providing the funds which attracted and secured for Duke the best medical staff in the region, it made the success of the other experiments possible. The willingness of the Duke doctors to invest personal income in supplies and facilities, secretaries and technicians, strengthened by common involvement the ties between the medical faculty and the University and greatly improved the service of the Duke Hospital. That willingness heralded the day when the members of the staff of the Duke University School of Medicine and Hospital largely assumed the financial responsibility for their future growth and expansion.

Chapter 6: Learning by Doing: The Training of Duke Physicians

James B. Duke left only two guidelines for the development of the Duke University School of Medicine: a general command to pursue excellence and a charge to serve the communities of the Carolinas.[1] These two objectives were not necessarily complementary. Ratings of excellence from the medical community at large depended less on producing able general practitioners than upon the contributions to medical knowledge made by Duke faculty and graduates. The need of the rural Carolinas for physicians demanded a rather different emphasis. The former required theoretical understanding of medicine, the latter a stress on the practical. For Duke the problem of what to teach and what to skip, common to all medical schools, was thus uniquely accentuated by the circumstances of its founding.

The liberal curriculum developed for Duke by Dean Davison on the basis of his experience at The Johns Hopkins presupposed that self-education produced a better trained physician. No formal curriculum, he reasoned, could include all the medical knowledge that would profit the student, nor could the school control the fields its graduates entered. Each, however, needed to gain a fundamental knowledge of the science and art of medical practice, and each needed to develop habits of independent study for keeping abreast of new knowledge and to increase his capacities for observation, comparison, analysis and deduction. Davison assigned slightly more than half of the student's time to acquiring that fundamental knowledge in required courses. The choice of additional studies rested with the student, subject only to the caveat that he demonstrate to the faculty that he utilized his free time profitably. He might choose elective course offerings, a personal research project which could earn him a bachelor's degree, independent reading in the library, or nothing at all.[2] Davison added one requirement unique to Duke: two years of internship or acceptable laboratory work before earning the M.D. degree. The student preparing for specialty practice or teaching normally took this training. The two-year requirement insured also that Duke graduates starting in local practice acquired seasoning in clinical medicine sufficient to make them above-average doctors.

The ideal of self-education and the eventual necessity of a doctor's being able to manage other persons made character and personality as important as intelligence in the selection of medical students.[3] An adequate intelligence was the basic criterion required to reduce academic failures to a minimum.[4] Each candidate from within a 200 mile radius of Duke had an individual interview with each member of the admissions committee. Those living further from Duke were interviewed by a regional representative. Candidates with generally poor records were not admitted, but a man with some low grades might be acceptecd if he impressed his interviewers as being personally suited for the practice of medicine. Those accepted received high marks for character and personality more often than for intelligence, and usually were described in recommendations as "industrious," "painstaking," or "hard-working."

A large majority of Duke's first medical students were Southerners either by birth or college, many from small towns or rural areas. One in four of those admitted to the first five freshman classes failed to finish his medical course at Duke. A few of these withdrew or transferred in good standing, but most were asked to withdraw by the faculty. It was not uncommon for students who withdrew from Duke to do creditable work and graduate from other medical schools.[5] As the national reputation of Duke University and its medical school increased, however, the geographical distribution of Duke medical students broadened, the percentage of rural students fell, and the percentage of students completing their course of study at Duke increased. By 1933, 39 states and the District of Columbia were represented in the Duke student body. There were also nine foreign students.[6] In general, students came increasingly from urban and semiurban areas; by 1940 rural medical students at Duke had dropped to four percent.[7] Students in the first five classes, required to present two years of college credit, usually presented three or more. As Duke gradually raised this requirement to three years in the latter part of the decade, two-thirds of the students accepted presented bachelor's degrees upon admission.[8] The percentage of students admitted from 1935 to 1939 who failed to finish their medical course at Duke was half that of the first five classes (see Table 1).

In college each student studied five or six subjects simultaneously; in medical school he carried only two or three each quarter. Alloca-

Table 1. Selection of students, Duke University School of Medicine, 1930–1939

	Freshman Class									
	1930–31	1931–32	1932–33	1933–34	1934–35	1935–36	1936–37	1937–38	1938–39	1939–40
Students registered	52	63	50	60	62	65	69	70	68	65
All or part of undergraduate education at Duke	14 (27%)	20 (32%)	21 (42%)	24 (40%)	21 (34%)	22 (38%)	43 (62%)	25 (36%)	20 (31%)	23 (36%)
Number graduated with Duke University M.D.	31 (60%)	44 (70%)	40 (80%)	44 (73%)	45 (74%)	53 (81%)	57 (83%)	59 (84%)	61 (89%)	58 (89%)

Note—figures compiled from student transcripts filed in the Recorder's Office, Duke University School of Medicine.

tion of teaching time to the departments in blocks allowed each student to focus his attention and to spend his free time on a limited number of problems. It also allowed the faculties of the various departments large blocks of time free from required teaching, which they could devote to elective courses for interested students, to research, or to other personal interests.[9]

The first two years were devoted almost entirely to the preclinical sciences: anatomy, biochemistry, physiology and pharmacology, bacteriology, and pathology. The primary objective of these courses was to lay a scientific foundation for the practice of medicine by showing the student the structure of the human body, the functioning of its processes and parts, the nature and effects of disease, and the effects on the normal and diseased body of food and drugs. The major secondary objective of these courses was to lead the students to acquire skills and habits characteristic of the physician. The scientific studies were designed to simulate as closely as possible the professional behavior of a doctor, so as to make the greatest possible impact on the student and to make the transfer of habits to actual practice easier. This strategy harnessed the student's desire to be a good physician to the subject at hand, thereby adding to his immediate motivation.

The heads of the preclinical departments shared a common educational method. The laboratory was the basic teaching tool, with the closest possible relationship between instructor and student the basis for direction and incentive. As the students worked at their laboratory exercises, the instructors acted as roving guides, passing from student to student to answer a question here or ask one there. Texts were mentioned as references, but specific textbook assignments generally were avoided, and the students encouraged to keep up not only through the use of standard texts but also through articles in recent journals. Only by familiarity with original reference material could they hope to keep abreast of a subject once the course was over. The importance of lectures varied slightly from course to course. In one they might cover the field in formal fashion, while in another they might only prepare the student for his laboratory work. In no course, however, were they as important as the individual experiments. Small group conferences, characteristic of education at The Johns Hopkins, were used also at Duke to develop close teacher-student relationships, answer questions about the work at hand, and evaluate each student's individual progress. These discussions sometimes ranged widely over the science and art of medicine, but through them, and their observations in the laboratory, instructors gained impressions of each student that largely determined whether the student passed or failed. No numerical grades were given. At the end of the course each student was discussed in departmental meeting and graded by consensus. Written examinations were given, but their importance was minimized.[10]

The medical course began in the Department of Anatomy, chaired by Dr. Francis H. Swett. A somewhat reserved Maine man and a graduate of Brown University, he had taught anatomy at The Johns Hopkins and was in charge of teaching gross anatomy at Vanderbilt prior to coming to Duke. His main research interest, which developed out of his doctoral dissertation, was in limb development in the salamander. Manipulating and transplanting the embryonic limbs and measuring the angles and extent of their growth required delicacy of touch, and painstaking attention to detail both in observation and record keeping. These same qualities he tried to develop in his students as they worked, four to a cadaver, dissecting first the skin, layer by layer, and then the body, section by section. He would pass from group to group, pausing to answer a question, sometimes entering into long discussions only distantly related to the work at hand. In these he communicated his involvement with his subject, and usually ended by leading the students to look again at their dissections to find the answers to their original questions.[11] In the afternoons the students studied the tissue structure of the systems they were dissecting under the overall tutelage of Dr. Duncan C. Hetherington, a Hopkins graduate who, like Swett, came to Duke from Vanderbilt.

Much of the first six weeks each year had to be spent accustoming the students to use their tools to best advantage. Often problems in this area were more the result of attitude than of ability.[12] A student disturbed by his first dissection might be careless and miss seeing the importance of a part of the body by cutting it away entirely. A student not used to doing detailed descriptions and analyses and unfamiliar with the microscope might find it hard to visualize cells in three dimensions. The junior faculty members, each of whom worked a quarter of the class both in gross and microscopic anatomy, referred major problems to one of the senior men. Hetherington found that relating a student's laboratory work to his future clinical practice was helpful in these cases. Describing a cell accurately was much like taking a patient's personal history, and required similar attention to detail. He sometimes spent as much as an hour with one student at the microscope, pointing out the errors and omissions in the student's description of a single cell.[13] Such tutorial teaching was expensive, in terms of faculty time, but it trained critical observers.

Dr. Swett and his wife, Elizabeth, who served as departmental secretary, were well suited to helping students through the stresses of their first weeks of medical school. With no children of their own, they took personal interest in each of the incoming freshmen. Mrs. Swett, a former grade school teacher, made friends very rapidly and could extract a great deal of information about their feelings with a few simple questions about dormitory life, food, or friendships. Dr. Swett almost never lost his temper and was willing to spend long hours trying to find the cause of a student's unhappiness.[14] If the student was bothered by the pressure of his courses and the seemingly endless detail of his assignments, Swett took pains to explain the importance of each item so that the student understood its importance to life and life-saving. If a student was working excessively long hours on an outside job to pay his tuition, he often found Swett arranging a loan for him. Dr. Swett is remembered both for the thoroughness of his teaching and the warmth of his friendships.

Next came biochemistry, presided over by Dr. William A. Perlzweig. Born in Leningrad, and a graduate of Columbia, where he earned the B.A., A.M. and Ph.D. in consecutive years, he taught at The Johns Hopkins for eight years before coming to Duke. When he spoke it was with a heavy, gutteral accent and this, combined with a mercurial temperament, kept his students on their toes.[15] Perlzweig taught the chemistry of the body and its products, particularly as the relationships among chemical elements revealed the presence or absence of disease. His favorite teaching device was to contrast normal and abnormal body states, and wherever possible he used the students as the subjects. After a preliminary review of chemical principles and experiments on the properties of carbohydrates, fats, and proteins, the students learned the chemistry of blood, urine, and digestion from their own bodies. They were put on normal, high, and low protein diets, swallowed stomach pumps, and studied the stages of their own digestive processes. Using their own blood and urine samples they learned the techniques of laboratory testing which they needed later on the wards.[16] "If they do it on themselves," he was fond of saying, "they will remember it."[17]

Physiology and pharmacology were taught as one course covering the normal and abnormal functioning of body processes, the effect of drugs upon them, and their effect upon drugs. Both Dr. George S. Eadie, chairman of the department, and Dr. Frederick Bernheim, in charge of pharmacology, held the Ph.D. rather than the M.D. degree. Accordingly, the course stressed theoretical rather than practical understanding. Students performed series of experiments showing the normal functioning of each body system, then introduced drugs to see how and why each particular drug affected the system and was changed by it.[18] Animal experiments allowed the students not only to observe these processes, but also to produce deficiency states and then treat them. For each subject, lists of current readings were supplied and checked on in small group conferences, the indirect give and take of which Eadie much preferred to his administrative duties, which annually gave him ulcers.[19] The students did not take up long lists of drugs as to their origin, specific utility, and proper dosage, as was common in most courses in pharmacology. Eadie and Bernheim agreed that the facts physicians needed to know to handle patients when their body processes went wrong were best learned at the bedside during the clinical years and internships.[20]

The preclinical professor perhaps most satisfied with the "liberalized" curriculum was Dr. David T. Smith, in charge of bacteriology. After graduating from The Johns Hopkins he had suffered a pulmonary hemorrhage and convalesced at a New York State sanatorium where, while a patient, he gradually took over control of the medical laboratory and studied non-tuberculous pulmonary diseases. This experience made him acutely aware of the close connection of laboratory to clinical medicine. He was given his choice of coming to Duke either as the professor in charge of bacteriology or as associate professor of medicine. He accepted both responsibilities in order to participate in the clinical teaching, which of necessity was the task given first priority in the new medical school, and to have ready access to laboratory facilities, where he could work to raise the priority given to research in the overall plan of the school.[21]

Dr. Smith taught bacteriology as a function of the department of medicine, using for his subject materials specimens from the Duke Hospital's central bacteriology laboratory. On the first day he gave each student two culture plates and asked them to leave one covered and the other uncovered during the class period. They began their laboratory study of the kinds of organisms which infect man from the cultures grown on these plates.[22] He was not concerned in his course to cover every known organism; rather, he sought to study thoroughly each group of organisms his class did take up, wherever possible using materials from the clinical laboratory and testing the students on their laboratory technique by giving them unknown clinical specimens for the same tests they would do on their own patients. Lectures, which, he warned students, did not begin to cover all that was necessary, introduced them to the ways organisms entered the body, the poisons they produced, the body's means of combatting them, and methods of preventing disease by active and passive immunization.[23] He then used animal experiments to demonstrate immunologic reactions and inoculation with toxin and antitoxin. A quiet man of scholarly appearance, he taught by example rather than precept, aided considerably with his students by peppery laboratory technician Mary Poston. Concerned not that his students know it all but rather that they know what it was all about, as a junior colleague remembered, he "just let it rub off."[24]

Dr. Wiley T. Forbus, chairman of the Department of Pathology, taught his subject both by comparative case study methods and by involving all students as clerks in the autopsies routinely performed by the department. For the first purpose the class was divided into groups of 12 to 15 and each group assigned to instructors in a room containing preserved organs, microscopic slides, and clinical records of cases grouped according to the type of disease. By comparing the numerous specimens of each type the students familiarized themselves with the appearance of the disease.[25] The availability of the clinical records accompanying each set of specimens helped to retain a sense of the individuality of the disease in each case, despite the use of the basic comparative method, after the example of Dr.

William G. McCallum, Forbus's mentor at The Johns Hopkins. As the groups of students rotated from room to room to study the different types of diseases the instructors also rotated. By the end of the course each instructor taught every group, thereby giving the student the greatest possible exposure to the experience of the members of the department and the junior faculty the broadest possible training in teaching.[26] A weekly journal hour, at which each student reported on at least one paper dealing with his current study topic, helped the instructors get to know their students more rapidly.[27]

The class was also divided on occasion into groups of three, each of which was assigned in rotation to attend autopsies. While the autopsy was in progress, one member of the group abstracted the clinical history of the case, one assisted in the removal of organs, and one obtained specimens and slides of the diseased tissues. Together they then prepared a clinical abstract, autopsy protocol (a verbal picture of the body and its organs and a description of the effects of disease on individual organs) and a provisional diagnosis, which they submitted before the report of the man who performed the autopsy was turned in for typing. To check on their work, students then attended the staff conferences at which the gross and microscopic evidence on the case was discussed.[28] Normally the students worked on at least three such cases, and presented the most interesting to the entire class for discussion in student-led clinical-pathological conferences, the most popular requirement of the course.[29] This clerkship in pathology gave the students not only an idea of the whole course of disease in an individual, but also a foretaste of the role of clinical clerk, which they would play on the wards during their junior and senior years.

How best to prepare the medical student for his transfer from the laboratory to the hospital was the subject of considerable debate among medical educators during the decade. With their hopes fixed on becoming physicians, students asked for and appreciated correlation of their laboratory work with clinical practice, but the occasional lectures and demonstrations by members of the clinical faculty only whetted their appetites.[30] The faculty, for its part, had to be satisfied that each student was prepared to handle patients. Proficiency in laboratory techniques was essential. In clinical microscopy, Dr. Oscar C. E. Hansen-Prüss taught the interpretation of what was happening in the body as revealed by its blood, excretions, secretions, sputum, and spinal fluid, using hospital patients for his demonstrations while providing complete hospital cases, with histories as well as specimens, for student experimentation. No student was allowed on the hospital wards until he passed a written examination and an oral quiz led by four instructors covering routine hospital laboratory procedures.[31]

Students also required practice in the basic techniques of taking a case history and doing a physical examination, the first steps leading to the treatment of patients, whether in the hospital or in general practice. The clinical faculty taught physical diagnosis on an interdepartmental basis in recognition of its importance, but Dr. Julian M. Ruffin was in charge of developing and organizing the course. The department of medicine took basic responsibility for teaching students the mechanics of history taking, and then the professor trained in each of the specialties lectured on the techniques of examining his part of the man. During each section of the course the class was broken down into small groups to practice these techniques on each other,[32] checking their findings by fluoroscopic examination. Gradually this course evolved into a complete introduction to clinical medicine for each student, bridging the gap between his experience in the laboratory and in the hospital. After the students were familiar with what constituted a normal physical condition, the department presented in turn cases illustrating common abnormalities encountered in the practice of each clinical specialty. Students practiced the techniques peculiar to each specialty on ward patients, and the laboratory knowledge of life in health and disease gained during the two previous years was correlated with the facts of each case presented.[33] By 1937 the course had come to require so large a block of time that it absorbed the entire amount of time available in the final quarter of the second year.[34]

From 1897, when Sir William Osler first introduced bedside teaching to the wards of The Johns Hopkins University Hospital,[35] the clinical clerkship replaced the lecture as the basic tool for teaching the art of medicine. Duke reversed the traditional Oslerian sequence and introduced its third-year students to the hospital wards, leaving service in the out-patient clinics for the fourth year. On the wards students saw fewer patients than in the clinics. The patients were selected to give the student exposure to all types of disease, an advance over the apprentice system, where the student simply saw whoever came into his mentor's office. In ward patients, diseases were usually more matured than in patients entering the clinic, making it easier for students with little experience to recognize symptoms and effects and to see the complete clinical picture presented by each disease. And on the wards the students worked less under the pressure of time, free to consult frequently with instructors and return to study the same patient.[36] As seniors, they worked as clerks on the out-patient clinics under conditions much closer to those of office practice: a steady stream of new patients, diseases in their early stages and thus harder to recognize, and difficulty in following up the cases.

Divided into three groups assigned to medicine, surgery, and the clinical specialties, the juniors entered the wards to take responsibility for the first time in caring for patients. In studying medical science and technology they had accumulated layers of knowledge about the body, its processes, diseases, their effects, and laboratory procedures. Each patient, however, was part anatomy, part physiology, part pathology, and so on. The art of medicine began by being able to take from each layer that knowledge which described the patient and piecing it together so that it showed what was wrong with the man and suggested how to treat him. The first skill essential to the doctor was diagnosis.

Each student learned diagnostic skills through a three-fold responsibility for each patient assigned to him. He took the patient's case history, did a complete physical examination, and was responsible for all of the routine laboratory tests, many of which had to be repeated frequently. In the first years, before house staff appointments were completely filled, the work load was extremely heavy. Dr. J. Lamar Callaway first registered in June, 1931 as a junior transfer student from the University of Alabama. One of only two students on the surgical service that summer, he remembers being assigned more than 20 ward patients as well as duties in the out-patient clinic in the afternoon. He made daily ward rounds with the surgical staff, and if anything unusual happened to one of his patients in the operating room he was paged and shown what the problem was and how to manage it. His work day began at 7:30 A.M. doing laboratory work, continued on the wards during the morning working up as many as 11 new patients per day, and in the clinics all afternoon. His day ended, after snitching milk or ice cream from a ward refrigerator, about 11:00 P.M. Living in the hospital in the interns' quarters with a private telephone line to arrange dates with good-looking nurses and secretaries seemed to offer a much better way of life than did the campus dormitories.[37]

The patients each student followed were the core of his medical curriculum. As in the preclinical years, textbooks were mentioned as references but not assigned, on the theory that the student learned more by approaching individual problems than by learning information systematically. The staff selected patients for the students to insure that each received a broad exposure to medical problems. This selection was expanded by the student's involvement both in instructional clinics and ward rounds.

The clinics, designated "wet" or "dry" depending on whether or not patients discussed were present for demonstration, were attended by all juniors and seniors and faculty from all the clinical departments and had as their objective a systematic coverage every two years of the types of medical problems commonly faced by the practicing physician. Although the clinics did not cover all the materials presented in the standard texts, the students could develop an outside reading pattern by being prepared to enter into the discussion of the cases presented. When the patient demonstrated was one assigned to a student, the student sometimes was required to present the case and be responsible for general questioning.[38]

Students were evaluated primarily on the wards, however, where the chain of responsibility for care of the patients served also as the basis for dividing the learning of the art of medicine into appropriate stages. Each student was responsible for the work-up of only a few patients. After doing the history, physical examination, and routine laboratory procedures he retired to the library with his problem where, with the help of reference materials, he organized his impressions. After talking these over with an intern or resident, he presented and defended his findings, and particularly his provisional diagnosis before faculty and fellow students the next day on teaching rounds.[39]

Rounds allowed more give and take than the clinics, although the tone of the rounds varied considerably according to the personality of the man in charge. The more sensitive rounding men usually began by making the patient feel as much as possible at ease. Then came the history, given by the student who worked up the case, emphasizing as much as possible the approach to the disease rather than details about the patient, and woe betide the student who was not familiar with the text and journal literature describing his patient's condition. Next came questions and answers in which the interns and residents on the service participated, and finally, if necessary, an examination of the patient and summation by the rounding physician. Then on to the next patient.

Each man had his own style. Hanes, the last of Osler's American interns to become chairman of a department of medicine, was a perfectionist. A southern gentleman of the classic type, he commanded attention simply by entering a room. The impression he created was captured by a brother of Dr. Hansen-Prüss, who drew pencil sketches of many of the Duke staff. All are fully detailed faces except Hanes's, which is a single bold stroke tracing the profile of his forehead, nose, and chin.[40] He would not go near a patient, male or female, whose axilla were not shaved in order to avoid body odors. His rounds moved briskly, for he usually felt that there was only one way to do a thing. He answered questions in the same clear manner that characterized his clinics.[41] Concerned always to preserve the dignity of his patients, he scolded no student more severely than one who was discourteous to a charity patient. The art of medicine, he admonished, knew only one class.[42]

The Duke University School of Medicine stressed the importance of a thorough general background for any field of medical practice, and Hanes required that his faculty demonstrate this to the students. Whatever his specialty, each member of the department of medicine was assigned to the wards and out-patient clinics in rotation and expected to teach from all the patients available, although he served as consultant on cases in his specialty. Dr. J. Lamar Callaway, hand-picked by Hanes to become Duke's specialist in dermatology, returned from two years of intensive study in this field at the University of Pennsylvania only to take his turn on the wards teaching students from all types of cases. The avalanche of new medical knowledge was only beginning to call into question the competence of the medical teacher to be a generalist.[43]

Dr. Deryl Hart and Dr. Clarence L. Gardner, Jr., his first resident who went on to join him in the department of surgery, were both very precise men. They had, as a rule, less routine exposure to students' questions on the wards because of their long hours in the operating suites. Hart felt the students on his service were compensated, however, because they had a direct check on the correctness of their clinical impressions through the operation, where the results of their provisional diagnoses were confirmed or contradicted.[44] Polite and genial, they were remembered by students not for doing any one thing in an unusual fashion, but for explaining everything so well.

Bayard Carter, chairman of obstetrics and gynecology, was a benign despot, "profane," as one junior colleague remembered him, "with a fine Oxford accent."[45] Always introducing himself as "Nick" Carter (no one called him "doctor") he kept up a steady stream of banter with his patients. Extremely gentle with a seriously ill patient, he was equally caustic with someone who would not make an effort to follow his directions, and not infrequently threatened not to return unless the patient disciplined himself more effectively. When he interrupted his joking with the patient to ask or answer a question, he did it quickly, and expected a similar response from his students. A poor suggestion as to course of treatment often brought the retort that such suggestions killed patients.[46]

Carter assigned cases to the students as they came into the wards, dividing the assignments equally between obstetrics and gynecology. Once a week seminars were held on the most common types of female disorders, hemorrhage, infections, toxemias, and endocrine problems, and on pathological specimens from operations. In addition, preoperative and predelivery clinics twice a week prepared the student for rotating through the operating and delivery room.[47] Much of North Carolina's population was not oriented toward hospital delivery and Duke, a referral center, handled a high percentage of childbirths with complications. To insure that each student assisted in an adequate number of normal deliveries, Carter assigned them for three week periods, under the supervision of a resident, to a prenatal clinic and home delivery service in Charlotte, North Carolina, run by Dr. William Z. Bradford. There they attended prenatal and antisyphilitic clinics, were on call for deliveries, and were responsible for four post-partum visits to each of 16 mothers they delivered on an average tour.[48] Every student, Carter felt, should participate in enough deliveries to acquire a sense of wonder at the beauty of the normal process.

Davison was the complete pragmatist. Well over six feet and 200 pounds, with a full round face featuring large eyes behind glasses and British guardsman's mustache, he appeared even bigger than he was. He lumbered into the ward on his morning rounds, shirt open at the collar, often without coat, followed by house staff and students, each carrying the portable camp stool he advised them to bring to sit at the foot of patients' beds and sometimes even out in the hall. Davison defined pediatrics as "general practice with an age limit of puberty."[49] The student saved time, he reasoned, if he learned adult medicine first and special pediatric facts afterwards, and in the latter years of the decade he moved the undergraduate pediatric instruction to the final quarter of the senior year (see Table 2). On the wards he rarely examined a patient. Rather, he took the facts as presented and engaged his listeners by describing clinical signs and symptoms as clues in a detective story and inviting them to arrive at a correct diagnosis, based on probability, by eliminating all other possibilities one by one as the clues suggested,[50] the method he outlined in the several editions of his popular text, *The Compleat Pediatrician*. Every performance was punctuated with illustrations from his previous experience in England, Serbia or Baltimore.[51] Only one third of known pediatric diseases were curable, he stressed, and these were at the core of his teaching.[52]

The routine work of the students, on the wards and in the outpatient clinics, was checked first by the intern on the ward. The internship provided the medical graduate with the clinical seasoning necessary for successful private practice or the broad background prerequisite to specialty training by giving him initial responsibility for the care of all patients on a single ward. Duke was the only medical school in the country to require the completion of two years of internship before it awarded the M.D. degree. (Seventeen other schools required one year.)[53] Despite a formal protest by the first graduating class in 1932 that the practice was not made clear to them

Table 2. The training of Duke physicians, 1930–1940

Course						Hours					
	1930–31	1931–32	1932–33	1933–34	1934–35	1935–36	1936–37	1937–38	1938–39	1939–40	1940–41
Anatomy (including histology & neuroanatomy)	429	429	429	583	583	583	583	550	550	550	550
Biochemistry	144	176	176	176	176	176	186	194	194	194	194
Physiology & pharmacology (including nutrition)	216	264	264	275	360	360	330	330	330	330	330
Bacteriology	88	88	110	117	119	119	150	150	161	150	150
Psychobiology	16										
Introduction to psychiatry							11	11	11	11	11
Pathology	288	288	288	397	396	396	396	396	396	381	381
Public health & hygiene										37	37
Clinical microscopy	96	96	78	112	121	121	112	110	110	110	110
Physical diagnosis (and introduction to clinical medicine, beginning 1936–37)	160	160	99	132	132	126	300	300	300	300	300
Medical psychology	16										
Preclinical exams	39	39	39	24	24	24					
Medicine (jr.)	286	308	308	308	308	308	308	385	385	385	385
Surgery (jr.)	154	308	308	308	308	308	308	418	418	418	418
Obstetrics & gynecology (jr.)						176	176	220	220	220	220
Opthalmology & otolaryngology (jr.)	110	110	110					66	66	66	66

Table 2. (Con't.)

	Hours										
Course	1930–31	1931–32	1932–33	1933–34	1934–35	1935–36	1936–37	1937–38	1938–39	1939–40	1940–41
Specialties (jr.)	198	308	308	308							
Pediatrics (jr.)						165	165				
Medicine (sr.)	286	286	308	308	308	308	308	391	391	472	472
Pediatrics (sr.)								191	191	191	191
Surgery (sr.)	220	220	308	308	308	308	308	309	309	309	309
Obstetrics (sr.)								120	120	120	120
Preventive medicine										22	22
Specialties (sr.)					252	301	301				
Clinical exams	39	39	39	24	24	24	24	24	24	24	24
Required hours	2,785	3,009	3,062	3,379	3,727	3,805	3,955	4,165	4,175	4,290	4,290
(%)	(54)	(58)	(60)	(66)	(72)	(73)	(77)	(81)	(81)	(83)	(83)
Free hours	2,363	2,139	2,086	1,769	1,460	1,382	1,193	983	973	858	858
(%)	(46)	(42)	(40)	(34)	(28)	(27)	(23)	(19)	(19)	(17)	(17)
Total hours	5,148	5,148	5,148	5,148	5,187	5,187	5,148	5,148	5,148	5,148	5,148

Note—the data for this chart are taken from tables in the catalogue numbers of the *Bulletin of Duke University*, 1931–41 inclusive. For a full analysis of this data, see below, page 124 ff.

when they entered,[54] only certificates were issued at commencement, to be turned in to the school after completion of two years of internship in exchange for the formal diploma.

The internship was similar to the clinical clerkship but with greater responsibilities. Duke offered only "straight" internships, confined to service in a single department, until the end of the decade, when a combined obstetric-pediatric internship of one year was offered graduates who planned to enter general practice. "Rotating" internships where the student served a short period of time in each hospital department, Davison felt, did not give enough experience in any one field to be valuable. Straight internships provided the best preparation for specialty training, and a combination of straight internships in two or three fields the most adequate preparation for general practice.[55]

On the ward the intern checked all the histories, physicals, and laboratory work done by the clinical clerks and worked up those patients not assigned to students. On call 24 hours a day, he was summoned to the ward whenever any decision concerning the care of a patient had to be made. If the call came at night, it was his responsibility to decide whether the course of treatment must be changed immediately. If the problem was beyond his competence, he woke up the assistant resident. This man, who spent three to four years in his position, was preparing for specialty training. Responsible for supervising more than one ward, he checked the work of students and interns alike, and handled whatever ward work they could not. In addition, he studied the basic science, auxiliary technology, and accumulated clinical knowledge peculiar to his intended specialty, and was given increasing responsibility for the care of patients at the discretion of the senior resident. Assistant residents in surgery also progressed through staged levels of responsibility in the operating room, moving to more and more complicated procedures.

The senior resident on each service made it go. Toward him the senior staff pointed their teaching most directly, involving him not only in their teaching rounds but in their private consultations as well. Selected for his ability to handle patients and students and to gauge accurately his own capabilities, he was responsible for planning the program for each of the assistant residents and interns. As the classes filled and the senior staff directed their teaching primarily at the residents and interns, the senior residents took more responsibility for the bedside rounds with the students, and made the results of operations and special procedures on patients available to students for study. They worked also with the faculty to set up the routine working procedures for the hospital wards. On the surgical services they were completely responsible for the operations performed on ward patients, and were expected to know when they needed help from the senior faculty. If a man couldn't tell when he needed help, he didn't get a residency.[56]

The end to every week in the teaching hospital came on Saturday noon at the clinico-pathological conference which all faculty and students attended. In the Hopkins tradition, a recent case, usually one involving death in the hospital, was selected by the pathology department and presented for examination. The clinical department involved presented a summary of the patient's history, the results of laboratory tests, and the course of the patient's treatment in the hospital, ending with a clinical assessment of the cause of death. The pathologist then presented the autopsy findings for comparison.[57] Often the two agreed but when they didn't, as Dr. Deryl Hart remarked, with wry understatement, "it added interest to the discussion."[58] In the open discussion which followed all aspects of the teaching of medicine, clinical and preclinical, were correlated in the study of a single problem. The conferences set standards of diagnostic evaluation and an image of medicine in its totality for the students. At the same time they served as a teaching device for the staff, first in the departments which presented the case and then in the faculty as a whole, which opened up and discussed new ideas and methods for future use.[59]

At every stage of their medical training, from first-quarter anatomy to fifth-year senior residency, the Duke faculty trained its students for responsibility by granting it. The education was a staged series of problems which the student worked at until he exhausted his competence and then asked for help. No single factor helped the system work more than the close personal relationships developed between students and faculty. The youth of the faculty helped, but the sense of sharing in a common enterprise, born of sharing in preclinical departmental activities and matured in the wards and clinics, was basic. The faculty members always were accessible. Laboratory or ward problems were often resolved over meals in the staff cafeteria. Invitations to visit faculty members in their homes came frequently in the early years, and students remembered pouring over Hanes's medical library, hearing Eadie play the cello, sipping homemade corn liquor after a round of golf with Davison, or enjoying an evening with the entire school at Josh Turnage's barbecue restaurant.[60] The same principle carried over into student government, which administered an honor system and could, on its own authority, dismiss a student from the school.[61] Students were thought of and thought of themselves as junior colleagues.

They were students as well as junior colleagues, however, and this was in part the cause of the failure of the "liberalized" curriculum to endure. They were, for the most part, not prepared to take full advantage of the opportunity to plan their elective work to best advantage according to their own interests. Many asked the faculty, "What do you recommend?" To answer this the faculty began to assess carefully the needs of the public for medical services and what types of experience with disease a man would need to meet them. And to implement their answers they began to think also of a more structured curriculum.[62]

The original curriculum represented the senior faculty's definition of the fundamentals of medical art and science and the time necessary to present these to the students. Each professor, however, knew much more that would be useful to a physician than he could present in the allotted time. Moreover, each new discovery, in every field, presented its claim for inclusion.[63] Small group teaching, coupled with the ideal of making the facilities of the medical school available to students whenever they might choose to do extra work, was extremely expensive in terms of teacher time. Research projects and personal interests were being curtailed. As the budget would not allow major increases in departmental staffs, some faculty members began to suggest that a more formal presentation of material would better give the students the proper amount and variety of medical knowledge and also allow the faculty to devote more time to research.[64]

The experiment broke down first in the preclinical departments. The students seemed to be acquiring an understanding of technical terms and the ability to recognize their importance from experiments. They did not, however, seem to be developing maturity of judgement because the block system allowed them no extended time to reflect on what they were doing. To meet this need the number of required hours in anatomy and pathology was increased and the courses spread over parts of two quarters rather than just one (see Table 2). Both Swett and Forbus found the increase educationally valuable, particularly because it increased the amount of contact between students and instructors and allowed more time in discussion for correlating the work with the student's plans for a career.[65]

Once the definition of training a good physician began to shift toward comprehensive coverage of medical knowledge, the departments and faculty members began, in effect, to compete for time to present their subjects more adequately.[66] Reexamining and striking a new instructional balance in the curriculum of the preclinical sciences eliminated for most students the possibility of a quarter entirely free for elective work, either at Duke or some other medical school, during the first two years. Throughout the curriculum, offerings originally elective but generally well attended, such as bacteriology's seminar on new developments in that field[67] and surgery's elective in operative surgery on animals,[68] became required. The content of medical education came to reflect relatively more the experience of the faculty and less the specific interests of the students.

No development better illustrates this process than the origins of the course in legal medicine. Soon after it opened, Duke Hospital was the defendant in a series of lawsuits for allegedly irregular practices[69] motivated in part, the faculty felt, by the desire of persons in desperate financial straits to enrich themselves at the expense of a large and seemingly wealthy institution. Out of the cooperation between the medical school and the Duke Law School in handling these cases came the conclusion that doctors and lawyers needed to understand the presuppositions and goals of each other's profession in order to work together effectively in medico-legal matters. On a voluntary basis, therefore, the schools began to cooperate in staging moot court trials in which medical students played the roles of expert witnesses and law students the part of opposing advocate. Questions concerning the case presented, and the roles, rights and responsibilities of each profession in legal matters, were then opened for general discussion.[70] The program was enthusiastically received by students of both schools.[71] Gradually the medical school made such discussion questions as the role of the coroner, the types of medical cases with legal overtones, and the relation of doctors to insurance companies and legal proceedings, the subject of formal lectures and, because such matters were a part of every physician's experience, required the course of medical students in their junior or senior year.[72]

During the last years of the decade the dismantling of the original curriculum was completed by the clinical departments. In the opening years Davison gave first priority of development to the departments of medicine and surgery, since they carried the largest share of the hospital's practice and earned most of its income.[73] Now, with larger volumes of clinical material and increased staffs, his own department, pediatrics, and the department of obstetrics and gynecology claimed larger blocks of teaching time. Simultaneously, the specialty divisions of the departments of medicine and surgery were developed by younger faculty to the point where they required more student time in class and clinic. By the end of the decade, the "free time" in the curriculum available to students was reduced from 46 to 17 percent (see Table 2) and the pressure for still more formal offerings continued from departments, and, within departments, from divisions. The competition kept the faculty constantly at work reevaluating their courses. Each new requirement, however, made it more difficult to add the next for fear of upsetting the overall schedule, and defining departmental purposes in line with institutional goals grew more difficult.

In the educational program of a medical school, of course, the example of the faculty and its attitude toward and interest in education are more important than the exact organization of the curriculum. The Duke professors were, without exception, specialists. As the medical school grew to full size more and more of their teaching time was directed toward the house staff, which itself grew from 16 in 1930 to 86 in 1939. Since almost half of the house staff during the decade were Duke graduates, they had a particularly strong influence on their fellow students, whose work they checked every day.[74] Duke offered only straight interships, and the residents were already involved in specialty training. As a consequence, the students rarely worked with anyone already in or preparing for general practice. Davison, in fact, felt that the residents made their preference obvious by encouraging interns planning to go through the residency and slighting those intending to enter general practice as soon as they had completed their internship.[75] Since most internships were for one year only, many graduates served as assistant residents before receiving their M.D. degree under the two-year requirement. More and more residencies were becoming available thoughout the country.[76] Moreover, a man who completed specialty training could expect to earn considerably more than a general practitioner.[77]

The Duke graduates followed the example of their teachers. Eighty percent spent more than the required two years in postgraduate hospital or laboratory training.[78] At the end of the decade, 56 percent of Duke's graduates were still in school. Of the 163 graduates in practice, 60 percent limited that practice to a specialty.[79] This was one of the highest rates of specialization among American medical schools. The rate of specialization for the total group of students who entered Duke during the 1930's was even higher. One reason for this, however, was that the many doctors in military service after 1940 saw that specialists received higher rank and pay. Duke had the highest percentage of medical alumni on active duty of any school in the country because, as a new school, virtually all of its graduates were of service age.[80] This experience distorts any measurement of the total percentage of graduates who specialized as a result of their Duke education.

Without question Duke contributed significantly toward making North Carolina one of the few Southern states which did not lose physicians relative to population during the 1930's. One or more Duke graduates or former interns settled in 37 towns in the state.[81] Duke graduates were more likely, however, to leave the state and the region than were those of other Southern medical schools. If Meharry Medical School in Tennessee is discounted because it was one of two medical schools in the country accepting Negro students only, Duke had a lower percentage of its graduates (30.7 percent) remaining in the state than any Southern school except Vanderbilt, and a higher percentage of graduates leaving the region (50.9 percent) than any school except Louisville.[82] Duke's student body was relatively more nationally representative at entrance, and the two-year internship requirement dispersed its graduates relatively more widely. Furthermore, the low per capita income in the rural South was not attractive to men with specialty training unless, as Davison continuously pointed out, they were born there.[83]

Hospital teaching was the first priority of the faculty of the Duke University School of Medicine during the 1930's because the faculty recognized the necessity of developing a broad clientele both of patients and students, the responsibility of the school to help improve medical service in the Carolinas, and the inevitability of being judged by the quality of its first graduates. Learning by doing was the principle which united the curriculum. The willingness of the faculty to try new methods, solicit criticism and ideas from the students, and assign meaningful responsibility made the students feel they had a real part in building the new school, thus heightening the excitement inherent in the experimental, case study, and bedside conference methods and turning the school's youth into an educational advantage.

In April of 1935 the last of the original wards was opened and the average daily patient census began to crowd capacity.[84] Four-fifths of Duke students were being accepted for more than the required two years of postgraduate training. With its clientele and professional staff growing and its graduates well accepted by the medical profession, the Duke faculty began to devote relatively more time to research, particularly on those medical problems peculiarly common in the Carolinas.

Chapter 7: Bringing the Laboratory to the Clinic: Patterns of Research, 1930–1940

The schedule of priorities set by the originating faculty of the Duke University School of Medicine placed research below teaching of students and care of patients in order best to meet the need of the region for a clinical medical center. This philosophy made virtue of necessity. No significant research was possible before patients came to the hospital in large numbers, the teaching load limited the research time available to any one man, and in the early years of the decade equipment budgets were gradually cut in some departments to as little as 30 percent of their original size.[1] During the depression federal government departments supported research at very modest levels. Neither did the private sector assume much of the burden. Pioneering private industries and foundations made grants to individual institutions and projects. Duke received invaluable research aid during the decade from such sources as Lederle Laboratories, the Rockefeller Foundation, the Markle Foundation, and others.[2] Generally, however, there was little money available to support research projects. Yet from the first it was accepted as axiomatic that a successful teacher, in order to keep his own spirit of inquiry alive and to develop a similar spirit in his students, must engage in original and productive investigation.

These circumstances determined the common pattern of research that was soon to emerge at Duke. A large majority of the research projects grew directly out of the medical problems commonly seen in the hospital and clinics. The dividing line beween "basic" and "clinical" research largely disappeared at Duke as the laboratory services and preclinical departments concentrated their attention upon investigating problems faced by the clinical staff and supporting their efforts to find practical, cheaper, and more effective methods of treating patients. Major research emphases were carried forward on an interdepartmental basis similar in its functioning to the pattern of cooperation developed in the diagnostic clinics.[3]*

* During Duke's first decade the medical faculty published over 800 articles and six books. This chapter can neither list nor assess each contribution; rather, it seeks to illustrate the ways of the Duke investigators, using examples which members of the originating faculty considered significant at the time, and especially those which contributed to Duke's growing reputation.

Since little medical research was being carried on in the South when Duke opened, investigation of diseases peculiarly common in the southern states offered not only the opportunity to contribute to medical knowledge but also to increase Duke's regional reputation. Endemic pellagra claimed the attention of the Duke staff from opening day. Pellagra became a major disease in the region beginning

Table 3. Deaths in North Carolina from pellagra (rate per 100,000 population)

YEAR	DEATHS	RATE
1922	330	(12.2)
1923	239	(8.7)
1924	281	(9.9)
1925	382	(13.2)
1926	455	(15.4)
1927	671	(22.2)
1928	851	(27.6)
1929	950	(30.3)
1930	1031	(32.5)
1931	695	(21.7)
1932	479	(14.7)
1933	392	(11.8)
1934	438	(13.0)
1935	383	(11.3)
1936	351	(10.3)
1937	332	(9.2)
1938	254	(7.3)
1939	205	(5.8)
1940	167	(4.7)
1941	144	(3.9)
1942	116	(3.2)
1943	105	(2.9)

Note—this data is taken from J. W. R. Norton, "Annual Report of Public Health: Statistics Section" (Raleigh: North Carolina State Board of Health, 1957), 85–88.

about 1910, when a gradual shift by farmers to one-crop cash farming (usually cotton or tobacco) reduced the average amount of meat and vegetables available per person per year.[4] The depression, which for southern farmers began at least three years before the market crash, simply accentuated these circumstances (see Table 3). Joseph Goldberger and his associates had shown that pellagra was caused by a dietary deficiency rather than an infectious agent. Pellagra could be induced by a diet of foods commonly eaten in the South, including white bread, corn bread, fat back, peas and beans, lard and butter, fruits, pies, and cakes. He found also that pellagra could be prevented by a diet which included generous amounts of lean meat, milk and eggs, and that a concentrated anti-pellagra factor was present in brewer's yeast.[5]

Goldberger died in 1929, however, without exhaustively investigating all the symptoms of pellagra, specifically identifying the anti-pellagra factor necessary in the human diet, or finding a treatment which seriously ill patients who were unable to digest large amounts of yeast could tolerate. Neither were his basic hypotheses universally accepted; some doctors still believed that deficient diet was only in part the cause of the disease. Several members of the Duke staff, including Drs. William A. Perlzweig and D. T. Smith and Mrs. Susan Gower Smith, had done experimental work on pellagra or other deficiency states before coming to Duke.[6] A practical cure for pellagra, they realized, would directly benefit the many Southerners who could not afford the adequate diet suggested by Goldberger[7] and would help to establish the reputation of the new medical school. Pellagra research, therefore, became a major emphasis at Duke.

Initial laboratory studies confirmed the investigators in their decision to follow the direction indicated by Goldberger. Negatively, Duke medical student Terry Wood found that a certain infectious organism thought by some doctors who disagreed with Goldberger's conclusions to be the agent which made pellagrins sensitive to sunlight was present also in the bodies of healthy persons.[8] Positively, Susan Gower Smith discovered that rats fed a diet similar to one on which humans developed pellagra contracted a dermatitis similar to one produced in rats fed a diet deficient in vitamin G (B_2), and that both groups of rats could be cured by the addition of brewer's yeast to their diet.[9] Subsequent experiments confirmed Goldberger's assertion that "experimental" canine blacktongue was an analogue of pellagra in humans,[10] thereby allowing the staff to test specific curatives on animals before humans.[11]

In the search for a specific cure, yeast was accepted as showing the dietary origin of the disease but rejected for practical therapy on the wards. Smith and Dr. Julian M. Ruffin, the primary investigators of clinical pellagra, turned instead to the use of liver extracts, which had been used effectively as early as 1920 in a pellagra-preventative diet but which did not become widely available for some years until they were prepared commercially for use in treating pernicious anemia.[12] Patients given daily doses by mouth of an aqueous extract of liver after three to five days showed marked clinical improvement. Patients treated intramuscularly with similar extracts generally failed to improve to the same degree.[13] These results suggested two hypotheses: that an element somehow lost during the preparation of the parenteral extracts was at least part of the pellagra-preventative in liver and that perhaps more than one factor in liver was therapeutic in pellagra cases.[14]

The pellagra research undertaken at Duke involved the investigators in some knotty problems of conscience and human relations. The histories of a majority of pellagra patients admitted to the Duke Hospital noted a generally deficient diet and a prolonged exposure to sunlight before the characteristic dermatitis developed, with other constitutional symptoms such as diarrhea, nausea, sore tongue, abdominal pain, and mental disturbance occurring individually or in groups in each individual patient.[15] The routine hospital diet with its abundance of meat, milk, fruit and vegetables, however, was a pellagra curative in and of itself. The potency of a curative could not be evaluated in a patient who was currently living on a balanced hospital diet. In addition, seemingly spontaneous recoveries from the disease were fairly common, although many such patients suffered relapses when exposed to direct sunlight.[16] Reliable research on pellagra preventatives, therefore, had to begin by placing patients on a diet deficient in pellagra preventatives.

Patients naturally would object to being placed on something called "Goldberger's pellagra-producing diet," so, with the assistance of Duke biochemist William Perlzweig and Hospital Dietician Elsie H. Martin a variant of this diet prepared for pellagra patients at Duke was labeled "Standard Basic Diet Number 1." This regimen was deficient in vitamin B_2 but was amplified with nutrients unrelated to pellagra. Pellagra patients at Duke were usually kept on this menu, without treatment, from three to ten days, during which the status of the disease was evaluated.[17] Those who apparently improved on the deficient diet were exposed to direct sunlight to determine whether the disappearance of symptoms was due to cure of the pellagra or to the protection from the sun resulting from confinement in the hospital. Only those patients whose symptoms were accentuated either by the basic diet or reactivated by exposure to direct sunlight were included in research studies. Such patients were considered cured when subsequent treatment produced prompt disappearance of all symptoms and the ability to withstand exposure to direct sunlight.[18] By utilizing the sunlight as a control factor the way was opened for specific investigation into the long recognized relationship between sunlight and pellagra, following Goldberger's hypothesis that the seasonal incidence of pellagra was conditioned by a high degree of dietary deficiency during winter months and the increasing intensity of solar radiation during the summer.[19]

Strict precautions were taken to see that these initial steps did not permanently impair the health of the patients. Ruffin and Smith visited each pellagrin every day to decide whether or not that patient should be continued on the basic diet and kept charts of each patient's daily progress. They agreed that if they differed on the course of treatment for any patient, Dr. Frederic M. Hanes, the professor of medicine, would be consulted, and his recommendation would be binding. As it happened, Hanes never had to be called in. Even with these precautions in force, however, the visible symptoms developed by patients were disquieting. Particularly unnerving was the case of a woman who developed a mental disturbance after exposure to sunlight. While disoriented she would cry "Oh why don't you take me to the Duke Medical School? I know they could cure me there." On one occasion some students even approached Dean Davison to ask that Ruffin and Smith stop experimenting on patients. Only statistical proof that the mortality rates among pellagrins at Duke were lower and recovery rates higher than among pellagrins on other forms of treatment elsewhere calmed their fears.[20]

Just as the Duke investigators, in cooperation with another research team at the Harvard University Medical School, were proceeding to isolate the curative factor from liver extracts to investigate its pellagra-preventing possibilities,[21] Elvehjem and his associates at the University of Wisconsin published a paper demonstrating that nicotinic acid was the element in liver which cured canine blacktongue.[22] The Duke staff was one of several groups which immediately reported successful use of nicotinic acid in the treatment of a pellagra patient, at a total cost of less than ten cents.[23]

The Duke investigators immediately applied the coordinated methodology of laboratory and ward studies developed during the investigations of liver extracts to research with nicotinic acid, and compared the results to those obtained from the liver research. Volunteer medical students were given large doses of nicotinic acid to determine its effects on normal individuals; their symptoms, charted for comparison with those of pellagrins, indicated that nicotinic acid was toxic and that large doses should be avoided.[24] Mrs. Smith and her associates fed various amounts of nicotinic acid to dogs suffering from canine blacktongue in order to predict effective dose levels for humans.[25]

Once the curative effect of nicotinic acid was established in the laboratory on dogs, appropriately scaled doses were administered to patients on the wards. With but one exception rapid recoveries resulted, whether the dosage was administered orally in solution, intramuscularly, or intravenously. The mortality rate among pellagrins at Duke dropped from 7 to 3.5 percent.[26] This dramatic effectiveness precipitated an entire new series of research projects which continued for more than a decade. Substances similar to nicotinic acid were tested as cures for pellagra.[27] This led to the discovery of secondary deficiencies which limited the effectiveness of nicotinic acid in some patients, and investigation of these replaced the earlier hypothesis that two or more factors in liver cured pellagra.[28] The investigators also examined the role of tissues and organs in retaining and excreting nicotinic acid.[29] Where Goldberger started the research which led to the cure of pellagra by reasoning from the pattern of incidence of the disease to its cause, the Duke investigators now began to reason backward from an analysis of the curative effects of nicotinic acid toward a more complete understanding of the substance itself and its importance for human life. Although these investigations and research on other deficiency diseases, notably sprue, continued, the battle against pellagra was won (see Table 3).

American medical research advanced during the 1930's in two general directions. One followed up the discovery that some diseases were caused by the lack of certain substances normally present in the body; the other sought to stop infectious diseases caused by living microorganisms.[30] The pellagra project was Duke's primary contribution to the first line of medical advance. Investigation of fungus diseases, particularly of American blastomycosis (Gilchrist's disease), was to yield a major success along the second line of advance.

American blastomycosis is an infection caused by yeastlike fungi which appears both as a chronic inflammation of the skin and in a generalized form which attacks the internal organs, presenting symptoms much like those of pulmonary tuberculosis. In its systemic form this disease was highly fatal. The same inherent logic which led to the investigation of pellagra led also to research on blastomycosis; there was a relatively higher incidence of the condition in the South relative to other regions and some of the staff had previous experience with the problem. In particular Dr. David T. Smith was interested in fungus infections, for he had seen, while doing research during his convalescence in a New York State sanatorium, numerous patients mistakenly admitted because local physicians were unable to differentiate fungus diseases from tuberculosis. He and his co-workers established two goals for their research on fungus diseases at Duke; first, to enable doctors to diagnose such diseases properly; second, to improve upon existing treatments.[31]

The first step necessary to insure proper differentiation of fungus diseases from tuberculosis was to make information on the fungus diseases known to general practitioners, so that they might turn to the laboratory for further diagnosis of generalized infections similar to tuberculosis. Descriptions of the different fungi and the methods of cultivating them for examination were presented both in national publications and local personal appearances,[32] based on cases seen by the Duke staff. Even with these descriptions, however, a bacteriologist not accustomed to working with fungi might well experience difficulty isolating and identifying them, especially if he did not possess the special tools required or if the focus of a patient's infection precluded direct examination of material from the lesions. In the case of Gilchrist's disease, since skin injections of the organism sometimes produced reactions in patients who did not have the disease as well as those who did and since the time necessary to grow and identify this particular fungus could be as long as three to four weeks, diagnosis was especially difficult.

In an effort to find a method for differentiating between the clinical pictures of American blastomycosis and tuberculosis, bacteriologist Donald Martin, who was recruited for Duke from the University of Rochester, investigated and established the effectiveness of the complement-fixation test in diagnosing Gilchrist's disease. This test measured the presence of antibodies in a patient's system by means of a chemical reaction with the agent in normal blood serum that combines with antibodies to destroy bacteria. A high titration, or amount of complement fixed by the antibodies in a patient's serum, generally indicated severe infection; a low titre or negative reaction usually meant that the disease was not widespread. No patients without the disease tested as controls reacted positively.[33]

Martin's work on the utility of the complement-fixation test as a diagnostic technique in blastomycosis cases directly aided D. T. Smith in treating the disease on the wards. The first patient suffering from Gilchrist's disease had entered Duke Hospital in December, 1930, complaining of pain in the chest for the past five years. Three previous hospitalizations, including one in a tuberculosis sanatorium, had left him only with the knowledge that he had a "pulmonary tumor of undetermined type." Smith's tests revealed the infecting organism, *Blastomyces dermatitidis*. He immediately started the recommended therapy, potassium iodide drops by mouth, but after initial mild improvement the disease spread rapidly and the patient died within two months.[34]

When Dr. Smith reviewed the journal literature on Gilchrist's disease, he observed that when a paper was presented by one physician describing the benefits of iodide therapy, often during the discussion of the paper another physician would report negative results with the same treatment. Although he continued to recommend iodide as the best available treatment,[35] the death of his first patient with Gilchrist's disease led Smith to seek some way of predicting which patients could be treated successfully. Eventually the similarity of the clinical manifestations of blastomycosis and tuberculosis led Smith to the hypothesis that the allergic status of the patient to the infecting fungus might determine whether or not iodide treatment would succeed.[36]

To test his hypothesis Smith began to test all blastomycosis patients, first with Martin's complement-fixation method to determine the degree of infection, then with an injection of heat-killed fungi beneath the skin to test for allergic reaction. Once a patient was found to be allergic to his infection, skin tests were continued until the vaccine was sufficiently diluted to produce no reaction. Beginning with that dilution daily injections were made, gradually increasing in strength. This procedure usually desensitized the patients enough to permit safe treatment of the blastomycosis with iodides.[37] Comparative studies of different strains of *Blastomyces dermatitidis* showed that they were similar in their antibody-producing structure so that a single stock strain maintained in the laboratory could be used to produce skin-testing material, complement-fixing antigen, and therapeutic vaccine.[38]

The case which finally proved Smith's hypothesis to his personal satisfaction developed from the misplaced zeal of an inexperienced young intern. A thirty-three year old man, generally in good health, was admitted to Duke Hospital with sores from which *Blastomyces dermatitidis* was isolated. Although his skin test was strongly positive, his complement-fixation tests were repeatedly negative, and iodide therapy was started. As it happened, Smith left town for a short time just after the patient was diagnosed, and the intern on the case, anxious to cure the patient before Smith returned, increased the dosage of iodides without testing for allergic reaction. The patient's pulse and temperature increased, his sores spread rapidly, and he began to lose weight (see Figure 2). At this point Smith returned, recognized that the potassium iodide was spreading the infection, stopped the drug, and began injections of stock heat-killed *Blastomyces* vaccine. Within a few days the patient's pulse rate and temperature returned to normal, he regained ten pounds in three weeks, and his lesions began to heal. Once he was desensitized, iodide therapy was started again and his sores healed satisfactorily. To prove that the patient's crisis had not been caused simply by sensitivity to iodides, Smith administered doses much stronger than those which earlier accentuated his symptoms and the patient tolerated them with no ill effects.[39]

Once an effective course of treatment was established, the Duke investigators turned their attention to the chemical composition of the infecting organism, the effects in humans of its chemical components, and to other fungus diseases.[40] During the depression decade members of the staff ran similar series of experiments, although less extensive, on other infectious diseases, notably brucellosis, a disease caused by contact with bacteria in spoiled animal products. These studies, particularly those on the infectious fungi, were soon to be of particular importance for American soldiers when the fortunes of war carried them into tropical climates, thus giving the Duke Medical School an unusual opportunity for making a unique contribution to the war effort.

Infectious diseases also were the most common problem faced by Bayard Carter and his staff in obstetrics and gynecology. The variety of these infections and the lack of knowledge as to their specific cause, however, led Carter to a pattern of research different from that of Smith and his associates. Since a wide variety of bacteria were found in the vaginal tracts of healthy women, it was necessary to describe the normal bacterial content of the vagina in pregnant and nonpregnant women before an infectious abnormality could be diagnosed. Numerous such studies had been made,[41] but the widely different findings were difficult to compare because there was no generally accepted descriptive terminology for classification purposes. Since the bacteria content of the average normal vagina varied considerably depending on the geographic region, therapy based on analyses made in other areas often was ineffective. Serious infections often were fatal: during the first two years at Duke Hospital the mortality rate among patients with infections in the blood stream following childbirth or abortion approached 13 percent.[42]

The only alternative to "shotgun therapy," or treatment with nonspecific vaginal medications in the hope that one would work, was to establish from tests on patients seen at Duke a complete basic pattern of normal vaginal flora. Vaginal smears and cultures from patients with infections could then be compared with the normal clinical picture to isolate the pathogenic organism. To the methods used in earlier studies Carter and his technician, C. P. Jones, added anaerobic culturing, which is to say a test for organisms which flourish only in the absence of oxygen. Studies were made on the vaginal secretions of 114 pregnant women and 100 gynecologic patients, including volunteer Duke nurses, who showed no sign of physical abnormality or vaginal tract diseases and who were receiving no vaginal therapy. The results, compared to those of earlier studies, showed a relatively higher incidence and importance in infections

Figure 2. Report of a case of *Blastomyces dermatitidis*

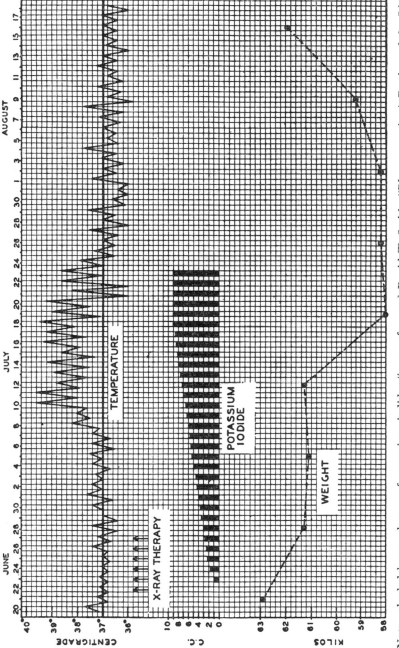

Note—shaded bars = dosage of potassium iodide (in cc. of saturated solution); temperature curve, in degrees centigrade, highest and lowest temperature recorded of each day; weight in kilograms. Figure taken from Donald S. Martin and David T. Smith, "Blastomycosis, A Review of the Literature," *American Review of Tuberculosis* 39 (March 1939): 296, and used by permission of the author.

of fungi and anaerobic organisms. These findings also established the necessity of careful preparation and study of anaerobic cultures before any accurate diagnosis of vaginal tract infections could be made.[43]

After identifying and counting the various types of bacteria found in the "normal" vaginas of the sample patients, Carter and Jones drew a composite picture of the normal vaginal flora against which to measure test results from infected patients. They paid particular attention to fungi of the genus Monilia (later Candida), for these frequently were pathogenic. They classified some 535 strains of Monilia into a system of six species, including a new specie, the stellatoidea, which they discovered.[44] Then they publicized their methods and terminology so that this basic bacteriology could be used as a diagnostic tool in other hospitals and clinics.[45] Once the fungi were differentiated and classified on the basis of similarities in appearance and growth, ability to ferment carbohydrates, serologic reactions, and pathogenicity in rabbits, correlations were made between their incidence and the clinical problems of patients so as to measure the relative pathogenicity of the several species for man.[46] Only after the doctors agreed on and classified, for communications purposes, what they were dealing with could the search for specific remedies begin. Mapping the medical battlefield was, therefore, a significant contribution.

Duke's endocrinologist, Dr. Edwin C. Hamblen, who came to Duke with Carter from the University of Virginia, followed a similar pattern of reasoning in pioneering the development of his specialty, gynecologic endocrinology. In 1931 little was known about the role of glands and their secretions in the reproductive process. Two discoveries during the 1920's, the demonstration that secretions from the pituitary gland controlled sexual functions and the isolation of the estrogenic substance now known as estrone from human pregnancy urine, opened a new field for medical research.[47] But what little was known left that field open to patent-medicine promoters and quacks such as Dr. John R. Brinkley, who rose to national prominence by 1930 in a series of radio broadcasts from a small town in Kansas by advocating the transplantation of slices of goat gonads into human testes to restore virility.[48]

When the first experimental and clinical trials of the new standardized specific sex hormones proved them effective, the Council on Pharmacy and Chemistry of the American Medical Association purged nonspecific ovarian patent medicines from its lists of approved remedies.[49] In addition, the Federal Radio Commission forced Brinkley to move his advertising broadcasts to Mexico, where he was beyond reach of the law.[50] Why the hormones were effective, however, was not clear.

The average doctor rejected Brinkley and his methods out of hand, but he also took a conservative position when it came to prescribing the new hormones. Because they were not well understood, and extremely costly, many local physicians were reluctant to stop using older medications which were substantially cheaper. "That is what I have to consider in my practice," one told Hamblen, "not to let the pharmaceutical houses get all of it, but leave a little for the doctor and not bankrupt the patient."[51]

Thus, when Hamblen followed Carter to Duke in 1931 he brought with him two key questions posed by the new discoveries: what reciprocal relationship exists among the organs involved in the female reproductive cycle, and how can the newly-isolated sex hormones be of practical use to the clinician? Reasoning that the hormones served as messengers between the organs, he decided to use the hormones themselves as the basic tools of his investigation. By treating patients with the hormones and observing any resulting changes he could draw inferences between the organ which was affected and the organ which normally produced the hormone.

Hamblen's method was limited by the availability of standardized sex hormones. The first two, provided in quantity by the manufacturers, were the estrogen, first isolated by Edward H. Doisy from pregnancy urine and produced in the ovary, and a lutenizing (follicle stimulating) hormone secreted by the pituitary, which also could be isolated from pregnancy urine. Therefore he began to investigate the relationship between the ovary and the anterior pituitary.[52] Doses of the hormones were given to patients suffering from a wide variety of disorders on the assumption that injections of these chemical messengers, supplementing or replacing those normally secreted by the endocrine glands, might help restore normal cyclic female functions. In each case the relief, or lack of it, as well as primary and secondary symptoms were charted.[53] Where relief of a problem commonly followed administration of a particular steroid, or sex hormone, Hamblen ascribed regulation of that portion of the menstrual cycle to the gland which secreted the hormone.

Given popular misunderstandings and professional misgivings, the first need of the new field was for order, and especially for description of normal function of female organs. Hamblen, a chemist by training, meticulous by habit, and more inclined toward laboratory investigation than clinical practice, was personally suited to this task. His goal was to describe completely the reciprocal relations among the organs of the female reproductive system so that functional bleeding and menstrual disorders might be recognized and treated in the clinic without undue risk of impairment of the sexual and procreative functions of his patients. The newly isolated sex hormones, which he necessarily used in treating his patients, were his investigative tools. During the day he took careful histories and made careful studies of the clinical symptoms of his patients before and after treating them with steroids. At night he studied the effect of these hormones on ovarian tissue, both animal and human.[54] By comparing the responses of his patients to the observable and measurable results of his laboratory studies, he could begin to formulate hypotheses about the normal female reproductive cycle and deviations from it.[55]

Once it became clear what was normal, the deviations seen in patients could be defined and described. Hamblen classified each case according to clinical characteristics, age at incidence of the medical problem, microscopic appearance of involved tissue and in some cases etiologic or causative factors.[56] His position on the staff of a medical center eventually allowed him to begin microscopic study of tissue taken, either in surgery or postmortem, from patients he had previously treated with hormones. Then he was able to describe the changes produced by steroid therapy and compare them with normal tissue to confirm or negate hypotheses as to hormonal effectiveness originally made on the basis of clinical observations alone.[57] He published his results not only as case studies adding to the sum total of medical knowledge but also as summary notes to general practitioners concerning the use and abuse of steroids in the treatment of office patients.[58] In establishing gynecologic endocrinology as a respectable new specialty he did not separate the roles of researcher and apologist.

Hamblen studied each new standardized hormone as it became available, observing its effects on the female reproductive cycle and incorporating this new information into his overall paradigm. The picture of the normal cycle allowed him to make useful clinical hypotheses. Having found that injections of estrogens would stop menstrual bleeding in the absence of ovulation and that injections of progesterone would induce it, Hamblen further theorized that administration of estrogens and progesterone in a cycle indicated by normal menstrual bleeding might raise the receptivity of the ovaries and endometrium, or the mucous membrane lining the uterus, to hormones in such a way that the normal menstrual cycle would be restored. When twelve patients given this treatment experienced regular cyclic bleeding and none reported a return of excessive bleeding after the injections were discontinued, the theory seemed substantiated.[59]

Hamblen's imagination in throwing out hypotheses and resourcefulness in confirming them won him a good deal of respect from his colleagues. As a consequence, he was authorized to set up a separate Endocrine Clinic within the Department of Obstetrics and Gynecology in 1937. Hamblen's classification system, based upon his own observations but incorporating the work of other researchers, now became both a paradigm within which the Endocrine Clinic staff studied each new hormone as a part of the total endocrine system, and a textbook for the guidance of other physicians and researchers.[60] General practitioners, with the aid of Hamblen's manual, could more easily recognize endocrine disorders and choose from among the increasing number of commercially available hormones the preparation most likely to benefit the patient. Reports of mixed results from physicians, however, indicated that not enough yet was known about how the organs effectively assimilated hormones to insure specific success. Studies on the receptivity of organs to hormones administered by various methods became one major line of new investigations.[61]

Hamblen's personal feelings sometimes dictated how he approached the questions suggested by his paradigm. The place of androgens (male sex hormones) in female hormonology fascinated him. Adolph Butenandt, the German physiological chemist who first discovered the presence of male hormones in the female reproductive system, had failed to invite Hamblen to help him in the follow-up investigation. Hamblen was piqued, feeling that his status in the field entitled him to the recognition of being included in the first group of scientists to investigate any such new development. He therefore began his study of androgens with the hypothesis that the male hormones were antagonistic to the normal female reproductive process.[62] Although he pushed ahead with studies on the source of these hormones in females, their function in the endocrine system,[63] and their relationship to each of the disorders associated with ovarian failure,[64] only after years of study did he grudgingly admit their possible therapeutic value.[65]

Compassion as well as injured pride, however, could dictate the direction of research. Although to many observers Hamblen seemed a taciturn and distant man, he was nevertheless acutely sensitive to the plight of the childless couples seen in the clinic.[66] Therefore he expanded his research on cyclical estrogen-progesterone therapy beyond the duplication of natural cyclical bleeding to search for an agent that would increase fertility. He tried several combinations of hormones, but the estrogen-progesterone therapy produced the best results. Four normal pregnancies occurred in patients soon after treatment.[67] Although Hamblen was seeking to increase fertility, later researchers built upon this knowledge, using the same agents in combination, to suppress ovulation by means of oral contraceptives.

Just as clinical needs shaped the direction of Hamblen's fundamental research in endocrinology, so too, in the Department of Surgery, a recurring problem in daily practice led to the major research achievement of the decade. As in other hospitals, patients at Duke who underwent radical surgery involving large operative wounds occasionally contracted severe infections, most commonly from *Staphylococcus aureus,* despite elaborate aseptic procedures.[68] Between November, 1933 and January, 1934, an "epidemic" of infections in supposedly clean wounds caused six deaths; as many in three months as had occurred in similar circumstances since the opening of the Hospital almost three years earlier[69] (see Figure 3). Careful study of Duke's aseptic procedures failed to show any flaw in the

Figure 3. Infections in clean wounds causing death, July 21, 1930, to January 15, 1941

Year	Date	Procedure	Clinical	Organism
1931	MARCH 21 / MARCH 27	EXPLORATORY LAPAROTOMY / CRANIOTOMY	PERITONITIS / MENINGITIS	HEMOLYTIC STREPTOCOCCUS, STAPH AUREUS / STAPHYLOCOCCUS ALBUS
1931	DECEMBER 22	CEREBELLAR	MENINGITIS	STAPHYLOCOCCUS ALBUS
1932	FEBRUARY 2	ARTHROPLASTY HIP	SEPTICEMIA	(BETA HEMOLYTIC STREPTOCOCCUS / B. COLI COMMUNIOR
1932	NOVEMBER 1	SECTION 5 TH. NERVE	MENINGITIS	SMEAR – GRAM POSITIVE COCCI IN CLUMPS
1932	JANUARY 12	SPLENECTOMY	PERITONITIS	STAPHYLOCOCCUS AUREUS
1933	NOVEMBER 15	THORACOPLASTY 1 ST. STAGE	PULMONARY EMBOLI	HEMOLYTIC STAPHYLOCOCCUS AUREUS
1933	DECEMBER 6	THORACOPLASTY 1 ST. STAGE	SEPTICEMIA	HEMOLYTIC STAPHYLOCOCCUS AUREUS
1933	DECEMBER 22	OSTEOTOMY FEMUR	EXTENSIVE INVASION	BETA HEMOLYTIC STREPTOCOCCUS, STAPH AUREUS
1933	DECEMBER 28	THORACOPLASTY 2 ND. STAGE	NO BLOOD CULTURE	STAPHYLOCOCCUS AUREUS
1933	JANUARY 16	RADICAL MASTECTOMY	SEPTICEMIA	HEMOLYTIC STAPHYLOCOCCUS AUREUS
1933	JANUARY 26	SECTION 5 TH. NERVE	MENINGITIS	HEMOLYTIC STAPHYLOCOCCUS AUREUS
1934	OCTOBER 31	SECTION 5 TH.NERVE	MENINGITIS	HEMOLYTIC STAPHYLOCOCCUS AUREUS
1935	APRIL 17	THORACOPLASTY 1 ST. STAGE	CHILL— / NO BLOOD CULTURE	HEMOLYTIC STAPHYLOCOCCUS AUREUS
1935	SEPTEMBER 16	CEREBELLAR	MENINGITIS	GRAM POSITIVE DIPLOCOCCUS
1935	OCTOBER 5	THORACOPLASTY 1 ST. STAGE	SEPTICEMIA	HEMOLYTIC STAPHYLOCOCCUS AUREUS
1935	OCTOBER 22	FUSION KNEE JOINT		BETA HEMOLYTIC STREPTOCOCCUS, STAPH AUREUS
1936	APRIL 20	CRANIOTOMY **	MENINGITIS	STAPHYLOCOCCUS AUREUS -- HEM. & NON-HEM.
1937	DECEMBER 9	EXCISION TUMOR NECK **	NO BLOOD CULTURE	HEMOLYTIC STAPHYLOCOCCUS AUREUS
1938 1939 1940				

*FIRST RADIATION UNIT IN OPERATING ROOM INSTALLED 1-15-36   ** RADIATION NOT USED

Note—figure taken from Deryl Hart and Samuel E. Upchurch, "'Unexplained' Infections in Clean Operative Wounds," *Annals of Surgery* 114 (Nov. 1941): 939, and included by permission of the editors.

sterility of instruments, linens, or supplies used in the course of operations, or in the sterility of the operator's hands or patient's skin. Bacteriological cultures taken from the walls and ceilings of the operating suites, however, did show the presence of this organism, as did cultures taken from the air in the rooms.[70] Either the organisms reached the operating suites from the corridors and wards, or they were growing on the walls and ceilings of the rooms, or they were carried in by operating room personnel. When daily washing and frequent painting of the rooms failed to lower the bacteria count, Dr. Deryl Hart turned his attention to the air, which since the days of Lister and his carbolic spray had been discounted as a primary carrier of contamination.[71]

The air used to ventilate the operating suites was drawn from above the hospital roof and "washed" by forcing sterile air through it; although tests revealed that this air was clean when it entered the operating area, staphylococci invariably could be recovered from the air when the rooms were occupied. Cultures of material from the noses and throats of the operating room personnel showed that up to 80 percent carried the organism, more frequently during the winter months, as was common among the population generally.[72] The amount of contamination was determined largely by the number of persons present and the duration of occupancy. Petri dishes of sterile blood agar exposed for one hour to the air in any operating room showed, upon examination, up to 150 colonies of pathogenic bacteria, predominantly *Staphylococcus aureus*. Clearly, it seemed, organisms in the air contaminated by human beings were responsible for most of the operating room infections.[73] To illustrate how potent the bacteria were, D. T. Smith and medical student Austin Joyner produced a powerful exotoxin which would kill a rabbit in two minutes, using staphylococci taken from the operating rooms.[74]

No method of exclusion or sterilization eliminated the organisms in the air. Personnel found to be carriers were treated with bacteriophage and antogenous vaccines until they were free of the organisms, all wore heavy masks over nose and throat, and limits were placed on the number of persons allowed in an operating room. Double doors were installed to separate the operating suites from the hospital, and the ventilating fans were set to force in more clean

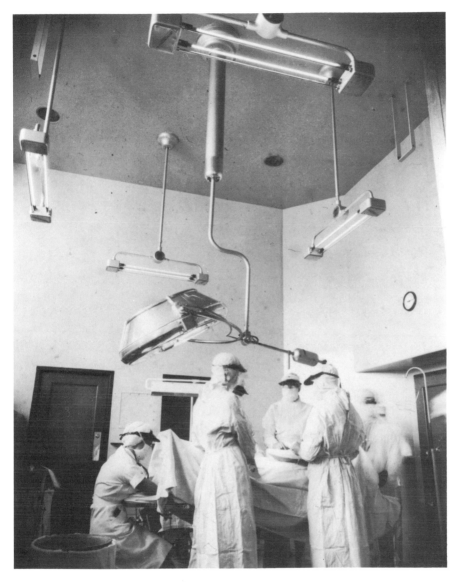

Dr. Deryl Hart and team operating in field of ultraviolet bactericidal radiation.

air than could escape out of cracks around the doors. Although the bacteria count dropped, infections were not eliminated.[75] Despite these and other precautions, because of the danger of infection the staff refused to attempt elective operative procedures of an extensive character during winter months. But this tended to retard the otherwise growing surgical service and to arouse fear of the operation in the patient and his family.[76] Somehow the air must be sterilized. There were, it seemed, three alternatives. An operating room might be constructed cut off from the rest of the hospital, with high-transmission glass for the walls and roof to let in sunlight.[77] Artificial sources of ultraviolet radiation could be installed in the rooms to kill the organisms. Failing this, immunization of all patients requiring surgery involving large operative wounds might be attempted.[78]

Only the second alternative was practical. There were neither funds for the first nor technology for the last. When experiments showed that rays from a therapeutic ultraviolet lamp killed *Staphylococcus aureus* at a distance of eight feet within sixty seconds, manufacturers were invited to participate in the undertaking. Eight lamps filled with argon, neon, and mercury, produced by the Westinghouse Electric and Manufacturing Company,[79] were arranged above an operating table. This device killed 95 to 100 percent of bacteria in the air and of *Staphylococcus aureus* at the operative site, in from one to three minutes.[80] Two blond student volunteers exposed to the rays for eighty minutes received only a slight reddening of the skin.[81] Experiments on wounds in rats and dogs exposed to the radiation showed that these wounds healed as well, if not better, than similar wounds not irradiated.[82] On the basis of these experiments it was decided to use the apparatus during thoracoplasties and other operations with large exposed areas. A protective dress of gown, hood, goggles, and eye shade was devised for the staff,[83] and the first operation on a patient in the Duke Hospital in a field of ultraviolet radiation was performed January 15, 1936.[84]

From the first operation results were striking. The radiation killed almost all bacteria about the operative area and supply tables, and up to 90 percent even in the far corners of the room.[85] Patients had less postoperative pain,[86] and the rate of infection in clean wounds dropped from 33 to 3.8 percent.[87] A patient operated on under the radiation was only half as likely to have a severe postoperative temperature,[88] and his wound generally healed more rapidly. Most important, the deaths from unexplained infections stopped.[89]

Hart's apparatus won the first award in competition with 107 other medical exhibits at the 1936 annual meeting of the Southern Medical Association;[90] thereafter it received widespread discussion throughout the medical profession. Among the first questions raised was whether or not the problem of the pathogenic bacteria was a local one, largely confined to Duke. But reports from hospitals in 17 states duplicating Hart's early culturing experiments showed the widespread presence of the bacteria in operating rooms during occupancy.[91] One of Hart's friends in a hospital where these tests were made reported that he knew his chief professor threw considerable bull, but he had not realized that it would be confirmed by culture.[92]

Once the extensive existence of the problem was established the discussion turned to the questions of danger and cost. Dr. Hart admitted that the possibility of chronic effects as a consequence of oft-repeated exposure to ultraviolet radiation could not be foretold, but his experiments revealed no immediate side-effects when proper goggles and gowns were employed.[93] The obstacle of cost proved to be negligible. An operating room in a smaller hospital could be equipped with lamps which sold at retail outlets for ten dollars each.[94] Some skeptics asked if Hart's results were not the result of general improvement in operating room procedures rather than radiant energy. The answer was unequivocal: the virtual elimination of operating room infections on different surgical divisions at Duke corresponded directly with the adoption of air sterilization by those services and the good results persisted despite subsequent changes in technique.[95]

Other surgeons gradually confirmed Hart's results. At the state sanatorium in the town of Sanatorium, North Carolina, the rate of severe infections in thoracoplasty wounds dropped from 23 percent to 1 percent using Hart's apparatus.[96] New England Deaconess Hospital, where a device similar to Hart's was designed and installed by William F. Wells, reported reducing the percentage of clinically significant complications in thoracoplasty wounds to 0.49.[97] Among Duke surgeons the fear of infection in major operations vanished. The major limitation on radical procedures now was the number of beds available.[98] Nationwide some surgeons doubted that the decrease in the risk of infection compensated for the increased discomfort while wearing Hart's protective dress during operations, but most agreed that he had shown what could be done to reduce infections in large clean wounds.[99]

Only in the preclinical departments which did not also provide major services to the hospital was research substantially separate from the problems of the regional clinical field. The work of the husband and wife team of Frederick and Mary L. C. Bernheim, for example, grew largely out of the circumstances of Bernheim's initial appointment. Trained as a biochemist, he was recruited from Hopkins by Eadie to be assistant professor of pharmacology. With no formal training in the field, he had to prepare his courses from scratch. The questions which came to his mind as he did this were those which arose naturally from his primary discipline, biochemistry.[100] Bernheim's first series of experiments, for example, sought to determine whether quantifiable relationships existed between drugs which produced contractions in intestinal tissue and those which would relax the contractions. His discovery of a quantitative antagonism between histamin and antropin was one of the steps which led to the production of antihistaminic drugs.[101] Comparison of this result with the action of other drugs allowed Bernheim to show which drugs acted on the same receptor substances in intestinal tissue and the amount of each drug necessary to produce the same reaction.[102]

What impressed Bernheim most in pharmacology, however, was that while drugs were known to affect the behavior of animals and to be affected by processes in animal bodies there was little biochemical knowledge of the interaction of drugs and cell catalysts, the enzymes which controlled the metabolism of the cells.[103] In this largely unexplored field there was room for experimentation with a large number of drugs, adding measured quantities to enzymes which could be isolated or to tissue suspensions to measure the rate at which each drug accelerated or inhibited normal enzymic processes, such as oxidation, in the tissues of various animals. Bernheim performed hundreds of such experiments, and the results of dozens were reported in professional journals.[104] He made similar measurements of reactions in which isolated enzymes hydrolized, oxidized, or reduced the administered drug,[105] and of reactions in which one enzyme acted upon another.[106] Each report began with a survey of the literature relevant to the proposed experiment, described the experimental process itself, and summarized the new data obtained. At the end of the decade Bernheim summarized his own work and that of others in the field in a monograph which laid the foundation for an entirely new series of experiments.[107]

Bernheim's work was a classic illustration of the process of test, report, and collection of data by which basic science feeds applied technology. Each additional experiment added to the total knowledge of the relation between drugs and life processes basic data essential to the production of safe and effective pharmaceuticals.

The feeding process by which basic research nourishes clinical practice was illustrated directly by Bernheim's next series of experiments. As the decade drew to its close the possibility of war increased and with it the probability of widespread malnutrition and a rise in the incidence of tuberculosis. With these threats in mind Bernheim turned his attention to the metabolism of the tubercle bacillus in an attempt to find a characteristic that could be exploited in a killing drug. In one of his experiments he noted that the addition of salicylate or benzoate to a suspension containing tubercle bacilli greatly increased the oxygen uptake of the organism. This suggested that substances of similar chemical constitution might play a part in the normal cellular metabolism of the bacilli.[108] The substances Bernheim studied were too toxic for human consumption.[109] On the basis of his results, however, Swedish biochemist Jorgen Lehmann tested over fifty derivatives of benzoic acid for bacteriostatic properties and eventually discovered that para-amino-salicylic acid was clinically effective against the organism.[110]

Work in each major research area at Duke began slowly and accelerated as the decade passed. This reflected the circumstances prevailing at Duke. Not until the medical school classes were filled and the course content set, and not until the hospital patient census approached capacity and the house staff grew accordingly, did the senior members of the medical faculty raise somewhat the priority assigned to research and publication.[111] A larger staff, and more important, an increasing number of grants from outside institutions, made this possible. Industry, private foundations, and the federal government began to fund research projects on a scale that eventually would take the primary initiative in determining the direction of medical research out of the hands of the investigators in the universities. The clearest early example of this trend at Duke was the work of Dr. Joseph W. Beard in the Division of Experimental Surgery.

Despite Dr. Hart's considerable work on air-borne infections, he did not look upon himself primarily as a researcher. As a condition of his appointment in 1930 he had asked that he be allowed to appoint a full-time salaried staff member to carry on research so as to balance within the department of surgery his own interest in clinical practice. Not until fiscal 1937–38 did three thousand dollars become available for this purpose.[112] At that figure he hired virologist Joseph W. Beard, a staff member at the Rockefeller Institute in Princeton, New Jersey who wanted to return to the faculty of a medical school in the South.[113] Beard was particularly interested in virus tumors,[114] and while working at the Rockefeller Institute with Dr. Ralph W. G. Wyckoff had successfully isolated the first small animal virus, rabbit papilloma virus, by ultracentrifugation.[115] Beard was to be in charge of a division of experimental surgery which would set up laboratories to continue his research on the physical and chemical properties of viruses and supervise research projects among members of the house staff.

Soon it was evident that funds were insufficient to support the technical staff necessary for Beard's work on virus tumors. Duke Endowment trustee William Brown Bell, however, was interested in Beard's work. Among the subsidiaries of the American Cyanimid Company, of which Bell was president, was Lederle Laboratories, a New York pharmaceutical house. Through Bell, Beard asked the Lederle staff if they had a practical problem related to his virology research which he might tackle at Duke with financial backing from the company. The Lederle officials suggested an attempt to produce a vaccine effective against equine encephalomyelitis, or "blind staggers in horses," a disease which was taking a large toll among animals throughout the world. Beard asked for $1500 to begin the research but Lederle Laboratories, realizing he would need more, made a grant of $6500. Reluctant to accept what seemed a princely sum for a project with uncertain prospects, Beard accepted with the condition that the unspent portion would be refunded if he did not produce an effective vaccine within three months.[116]

Beard could set so rigid a timetable for the project only because he was already familiar with the technology necessary for the experiment. It was known that injections of noninfectious formalin-treated brains of horses or guinea pigs dying of this disease would protect healthy horses or guinea pigs against injections of the active virus. Although healthy animals tended to reject vaccine grown in tissues of other animals, the virus could be grown in high concentration in chick embryos, and the Duke investigator thought it might be possible to isolate the virus from them to make a pure vaccine.[117] Beard's colleague at the Rockefeller Institute, R. W. C. Wyckoff, had recently isolated the virus responsible for equine encephalomyelitis by ultracentrifugation.[118] Beard proposed simply to grow the virus in chick embryos, purify it by ultracentrifugation, kill it with formaldehyde, and inoculate guinea pigs with the pure vaccine. The effectiveness of the vaccine then could be tested by injecting live virus into the animals. Only the killing of the virus was difficult; too much formaldehyde would destroy the virus and too little would not kill it all.

Three groups of animals were used in the experiments. One group got no medication. One was injected with the pure vaccine. The third received, as a control, a crude vaccine made up of formaldehyde-treated diseased chick embryos in ten percent solution. Soon after their inoculation, all were infected with the active virus.[119] Although all the guinea pigs treated with the pure vaccine lived longer than those treated with live virus alone, some did die later from the toxic effects of the concentrated formaldehyde. To the astonishment of Beard and his associates, however, all of the guinea pigs treated with the crude vaccine lived, remaining immune to the live virus. Not only was the crude vaccine more effective, it was cheaper to produce since it took fewer infected embryos to make each dose and since the expensive process of getting the virus out of the embryos was eliminated.[120] Immediately the results were rushed to Lederle Laboratories, where tests proved the vaccine was equally effective in horses.[121] The entire project, begun in early October, 1937, was essentially completed before Christmas.

Lederle Laboratories patented the vaccine in Beard's name, with five percent of the gross profits to be donated to Duke University. At the suggestion of University counsel E. W. Bryson these funds, amounting to over $38,000 in the first year alone, were placed in a separate account known as the Dorothy Beard Research Fund. Administered by Beard, Davison and Hart, this fund was used not only to support the research projects of Beard's staff but also to make interest-free loans to faculty members building homes in the community and for departmental purposes. Lederle Laboratories thereafter continued to make annual grants for the support of the work of Beard's division.[122]

Within months after the vaccine went into production a research team at Harvard discovered that the equine encephalomyelitis virus could be fatal to man.[123] Immediately Beard was called to New York to examine the Lederle Laboratory workers. Among them, and among his own staff, a high percentage were infected with the virus, one-third of the first group of 69 tested.[124] Using a vaccine prepared in the same way as that used in horses but only forty percent of the horse dosage and effective against both known strains of the disease, Beard vaccinated both the staff at Lederle Laboratories and the members of the Duke staff who had worked with the vaccine. This immunization marked the first successful use of killed-virus vaccine in humans.[125]

Except for the brief flurry of work related to human immunization, the equine encephalomyelitis vaccine project ended at Duke in January, 1938. With the financial support attracted from Lederle Laboratories, the National Cancer Institute, and other outside agencies, Beard and his staff returned to and expanded their work on the physical and chemical properties of the equine encephalomyelitis, papilloma, and other viruses, and the effects of these viruses on animals. With the coming of war, however, they returned to vaccine research and production at the request of the U.S. Army.[126]

Research at Duke during the depression decade was determined first, by the incidence of problems in the clinical field; second, by the personal interests and previous experience of individual investigators; third, by the stage of development of the hospital and medical school; fourth, by the availability of funds. The agreed-upon priorities established to build the medical school and hospital and the lack of funds from outside Duke University dictated that this should be so. In large part the research was supported by the professors themselves, in the sense that they did not render accounting to anyone for their time or for many minor expenses. Although each project was primarily associated with the names of one or two men, most investigative efforts were interdepartmental. The most common pattern found the preclinical departments which also rendered analytical service to hospital patients, including Bacteriology, Pathology, and Biochemistry, working with the clinical departments to find the cause of problems seen on the wards.

In this process the research initiative lay primarily with the investigators. Smith and Ruffin sought to increase medical knowledge and at the same time the reputation of the new school by eradicating diseases peculiarly southern. Carter and Hamblen sought to establish norms by which to isolate, measure, and treat gynecologic diseases. Hart eliminated one source after another as the medium of infections in his operating room. But all of these rational designs were grounded in the circumstances of their medical practice. The secondary determinants also were personal: Smith's previous experience with fungus diseases, Bernheim's biochemical approach to pharmacology, or Hamblen's compassion for childless couples and his resentment toward Butenandt for neglecting him. Each man was largely free to solicit funds for his projects where he could and to use them as he would.

Beard's virology projects, however, were a foretaste of the future. His search for an effective vaccine against equine encephalomyelitis, bought and paid for by Lederle Laboratories, showed the kind of rapid progress possible if adequate funds were available. This was especially evident when, as a result of Beard's project, Lederle Laboratories and the National Cancer Institute continued to support work along related lines. As war clouds gathered, the needs of the military made research a national resource. The Beard group's production of human vaccines was only one of hundreds of projects at universities bought and paid for by the government. As the larger funds of government, industry, and foundations were marshalled in support of scientific research, they also helped to set its goals.[127] After the war the groups of university professors who passed on projects submitted for funding to the National Institutes of Health would be especially influential in developing broad guidelines for American medical research. The universities themselves, however, continued to be the basic research agencies.

Chapter 8: Modernizing Medical Care: Cooperation with The Duke Endowment

The primary objective of James B. Duke's philanthropy was to improve the quality of medical care throughout the Carolinas. He believed that only the people could bear financial responsibility for so great a problem, and he directed the largest portion of his benevolences to helping the people to accept that responsibility.[1]

As Dr. Watson S. Rankin, Director of the Hospital Section of The Duke Endowment, had explained the problem to him, adequate medical care rested on a tripod of services: physicians in adequate numbers throughout the area, hospital facilities, and nursing and technical personnel. Providing hospital facilities in rural areas was the best means of assuring all three. Hospitals attracted newly-graduated doctors by giving them opportunities to utilize their skills fully. Hospitals also attracted the nurses and technicians who multiplied the doctors' skills by their own. Finally, hospitals eliminated the waste of time then being consumed in traveling from one patient to another.[2]

The Duke University School of Medicine and Hospital cooperated with The Duke Endowment in its mission of modernizing medical care in the Carolinas. For its part The Duke Endowment utilized three primary devices. First, it supported the operating budgets of hospitals to the extent of one dollar per patient day of free care given by the hospitals, thereby increasing the number of Carolinians receiving adequate treatment. By 1929 the total number of patient days of care given by assisted hospitals rose 70 percent, most of the increase being free care given to the poor. Second, The Endowment provided the hospitals it assisted with statistical analyses of their medical and administrative operations compared to those of other similar hospitals. Using the average achievements of assisted hospitals as standards, Endowment staff members were able to identify for individual hospitals areas where their costs were too high and to suggest less expensive or more efficient procedures. Between 1925 and 1929 the average per diem cost of hospitalization to patients in assisted hospitals did not rise, due in part to economies suggested by The Duke Endowment.[3] Third, the Hospital Section expended any surplus funds in aiding communities to build or equip new hospitals. In most instances The Endowment required the local community to raise from one-half to two-thirds of the necessary capital before contributing the balance.[4] By 1931, The Endowment assisted in the construction of 25 new hospitals, the improvement of 21, and the purchase of 10 from private owners.[5] A revolution in the form of a dramatic shift from private to public responsibility for health services was well underway.

In addition to training doctors, the Duke University School of Medicine and Hospital cooperated with The Endowment in four major areas. Training programs in health service professions provided the nurses, technicians, and administrators needed in new modern hospitals. When the statistical analyses of The Duke Endowment revealed inadequacies in professional care given by an individual hospital, members of the Duke faculty served as consultants in improving conditions. Also, the Department of Pathology operated an outside pathological service which reviewed the necessity and effectiveness of all surgical procedures performed in subscribing hospitals. Finally, the annual Duke University three-day Medical Symposia offered the region's general practitioners regular opportunities to refurbish their skills.

In effect, the relationship between The Duke Endowment and the School of Medicine and Hospital was reciprocal. The number and variety of patients seeking treatment at Duke increased to a considerable extent because of the influence of the public officials, private citizens, and local physicians identified with the local hospitals assisted by The Duke Endowment. The Duke Hospital and Medical School repaid the Carolinas for their clinical material with the trained manpower needed to modernize the region's medical care.

The School of Nursing was by far the largest of Duke's training programs in the health service professions. As the only school in North Carolina associated with a university as well as a hospital, Duke hoped to attract into nursing girls meeting the same entrance requirements of intelligence, character, and high school preparation as those admitted to the women's college of the University. The social and recreational opportunities offered by the University were

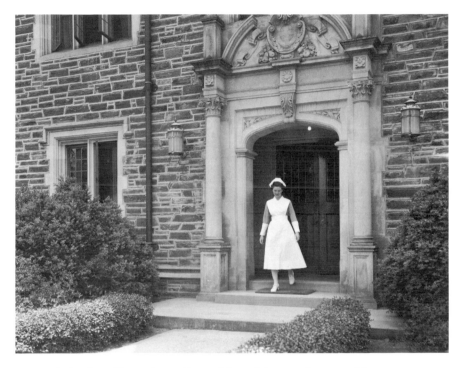

A Student Nurse in uniform, Nurses' Home doorway, May, 1941

prominently featured in promotional literature.[6] For the girl who wished only to prepare for professional work a basic three-year program led to the Diploma of Graduate Nurse. But for the girl who wished a college degree as well, Duke University offered the Bachelor of Science in Nursing to candidates who presented 60 hours of college work taken either before or after, but not during, the basic nursing program. Students in the five-year program were offered the choice of preparing directly for teaching in schools of nursing, supervisory nursing positions, or public health nursing.[7]

Girls in degree programs, however, took exactly the same basic nursing course as diploma candidates. During the first six months, a probationary period, the accent was placed on academics. Lectures and laboratory experience in anatomy, chemistry, bacteriology, pharmacy, and nutrition, taught by members of the Duke medical faculty and Miss Anne Gardiner, who as Assistant Professor of Nursing Education taught or assisted with most of the courses in the School of Nursing, took most of the student's time. This classwork took its toll. Of 42 pupil nurses admitted in 1937, for example, nine resigned during the probationary period either because they felt they could not carry the work or because they had come to dislike nursing.[8]

After the probationary period, training was almost entirely practical. Nursing like medicine, according to Dean Davison, was best learned by "doing," complemented by a sufficient understanding of the methods used to enable the nurse to assist the physician effectively.[9] Each girl worked 52 hours weekly on the wards compared with an average of eight in the classroom. Most of the lectures during the last two years acquainted the nurses with the problems and procedures peculiar to the service on which they were working.[10] Students rotated through each of the departments of the hospital, including the clinics. The test of the student's knowledge was her performance on the wards. One error might bring a reprimand; three might result either in her being asked to repeat the appropriate course or even dropped from the school.[11] One of every ten students admitted during the first seven years left school for personal reasons; four in ten were dropped by the school.[12] The rigor of the course, however, helped keep morale high among those who succeeded.[13] Almost half of those who graduated went on to take a bachelor's degree,[14] and one-third remained at Duke Hospital to practice.[15]

The self-image of the nurse began to change, however, during the 1930's. Women accredited through long hours of ward practice in hospital schools of nursing generally defined their profession in terms of sensitivity to the needs of others, caring for patients, and aiding the physician at his work. As the complexity of and time required for diagnostic, therapeutic, and surgical procedures increased, busy clinicians began to turn more and more of these procedures over to graduate nurses.[16] As demands upon their skills increased, nurses and especially national nursing organizations began to define their vocation more in terms of cultural and professional competence and less, if only relatively, in terms of hospital service. The collegiate school of nursing replaced the hospital school as the ideal, if not the norm. A shorter work week, a greater range of elective courses with a greater number of courses in the liberal arts to develop the nurse as an individual and citizen, and a voice for the nurse in the government of her school all became new professional goals.[17] The Association of Collegiate Schools of Nursing required for approval that a university school of nursing have a similar organization to that of other professional schools; that is, that it be under the direct control of the university rather than the university hospital.[18]

Nursing students at Duke, encouraged by the medical and nursing faculties, elected the five-year degree program in increasing numbers.[19] Since statistical analyses of Duke student nurses showed that scholastic failures decreased and psychological maturity increased with the number of years of college preparation,[20] the admissions committee sought especially girls who had completed at least two years. On paper the goals and curriculum of the Duke school were identical with national standards.

Duke was, however, essentially a hospital school grafted onto a university structure. Dean Davison believed in the university-type schools as attracting and liberal arts courses as producing a better quality of nurse, but he and other members of the staff also valued the personal sensitivity and dedication of nurses trained primarily in the hospital.[21] The nursing faculty generally did not rank with the university faculty in terms of professional preparation and because of limited budgets were few in number compared to the staffs of other university-type nursing schools.[22] Since the turnover rate of graduate nurses, three times that of any other employee category, was forcing the hospital to hire increasing numbers of untrained and correspondingly inefficient personnel, Davison could see his way clear neither to reduce the student-service contribution below 52 hours weekly nor to relinquish control of the school of nursing.[23]

The choice between national standards and local conditions offered three alternatives: to meet national requirements, to disregard the Association of Collegiate Schools of Nursing while continuing to offer a degree program, or to become a hospital school only.[24] The high rating placed by Duke's senior medical faculty on nursing skills learned at the bedside and a lack of funds for hiring nurses to staff new additions to the hospital, which made the student-service contribution on the wards even more valuable,[25] decided the issue in favor of the hospital school alternative. The degree program was discontinued.[26] Duke withdrew from the Association of Collegiate Schools of Nursing, the nursing school remained a department of the School of Medicine, and instruction of nurses became the direct care of the departments in which they worked, together with the small nursing faculty.[27] Almost a decade passed before Duke considered returning to the concept of a degree-offering university school of nursing.

The same emphasis on practical experience characterized the Duke training programs for other types of hospital personnel, notably dietitians, administrators, and technicians. Both Dean Davison and Professor of Medicine Harold L. Amoss were anxious to establish a school for dietitians, Amoss because of the importance of dietary control in many medical treatments, and Davison to meet the growing need of hospitals in the Carolinas. No school in the South offered a full year's training in dietetics, although Watts Hospital in Durham offered an accredited six-month program. Both Davison and Amoss also shared the belief that opportunity to understand the clinical background of diet work should be the heart of the program.[28]

The standards of the new profession of dietetics were still in the process of definition. The American Dietetic Association required members to hold a bachelor's degree with a major in foods or nutrition and a graduate program of at least six months, including administrative practice, diet therapy, and teaching of student nurses.[29] Dean Davison and Professor of Dietetics Elsie Martin agreed that a full year of training was preferable. Davison feared, however, that the most well qualified students might not wish to invest more time than necessary in graduate training. He therefore arranged for Duke University to offer a bachelor's degree to women who completed three and one-half years of college, including the major in foods or nutrition, and a one year program in dietetics at Duke. As in the case of the medical curriculum, he preferred to shorten college preparation in favor of increased clinical experience.[30] The American Dietetic Association soon required a full year of graduate training, however, and the provision for shortening college preparation was dropped.[31]

The American Dietetic Association approved the Duke program as soon as the Duke Hospital patient census met Association requirements. Student dietitians studied biochemistry, nutrition, and physiology alongside the medical students and accompanied the medical staff on ward rounds to study cases involving a relationship between diet and disease. In addition, the dietetic interns rotated through the several kitchens of the Duke Hospital, taking responsibility for organizing equipment, computing and serving special diets, planning menus, purchasing food, and supervising the entire operation of the main Duke kitchen. In addition, they taught both student nurses and families of patients how to prepare and serve the special diets prescribed by doctors. Each student was evaluated as to her personality, skill with foods, administrative ability and teaching effectiveness,[32] and recommendations to potential employers made accordingly.

For laboratory technicians, in contrast to the situation in dietetics, no accrediting agency existed in 1930. From the opening of Duke Hospital each faculty member had to recruit these workers wherever he could and train them, whenever he had time, on an apprenticeship basis. This individual instruction produced excellent technicians,[33] but required a great deal of time from the medical faculty, did not produce a steady supply of technicians, and was difficult for other hospitals to evaluate when Duke-trained people applied for positions elsewhere. To meet these problems Susan Gower Smith, Donald Martin, and Haywood Taylor organized a formal training program in laboratory technique in 1932, open to students with two years of college preparation with credits in basic science equivalent to those of entering medical students.

The eighteen-month program placed the same stress on practical experience as did the curricula in nursing and dietetics, hours at work in the laboratory outnumbering hours spent in lectures 25 to 1.[34] Students rotated through the laboratories of each major medical service to learn their procedures on the job. The technician in charge of the laboratory kept records of the procedures each student mastered, and these were noted on his transcript as a guide to future employers.[35] Student technicians took the same lectures and laboratory work as the medical students in such fields as hematology and bacteriology, and also attended the clinical pathological conferences. Other courses, such as blood chemistry, met the special needs of technicians.[36] By the end of the decade some 60 students, almost all either born or educated in the South, completed the program. Demand for their services far exceeded the supply, even without advertising their availability.[37]

The hospital program of The Duke Endowment created demand not only for nurses and technicians to multiply the doctor's skills, but also for hospital administrators trained to keep operating expenses at a minimum and medical service at a maximum. In the average hospital the administrator allocated funds, supervised the business operations, harmonized interdepartmental relationships, recruited staff, decided who was eligible for charity care, represented the hospital before the local community, and prepared the records necessary for participation in the Endowment's statistical information service. Yet most administrators were doctors or nurses who drifted into the field from local necessity but with no specialized training for the role. One in five was a layman who brought business experience, but little knowledge of problems unique to hospitals, to his job. Nowhere in the country were administrators being trained specifically to work in hospitals.[38] In a study made for the Rockefeller Foundation just before the Duke Hospital opened its doors, medical economist Michael M. Davis pointed to the need for a training center for hospital administrators at a major university, with a curriculum centered in on-the-job experience which would train administrative interns to adapt business methods to the network of medical, personal, and community relations in the hospital so as to serve patients more efficiently.[39]

Inspired by Davis's thesis and the need for trained administrators both at Duke and in the institutions assisted by The Duke Endowment, Dean Davison instituted the first graduate course in the country to meet this requirement when Duke Hospital opened in 1930. The new program accepted graduates in business administration for a two year combination of orientation in the health and hospital field and application of administrative principles to hospital problems. The administrative interns were given supervisory responsibility in the administrative areas of the hospital on a rotating basis, beginning with opening boxes of equipment in the hospital basement. They also met with Dean Davison once a week for discussions on how to relate previous academic experience to current management problems. Operating procedures were learned by rule of thumb. Davison also hoped that his administrative interns would educate the medical, surgical and other residents and interns who lived with them in the unused hospital rooms which doubled as the house staff quarters to the problems of hospital management. This would, he felt, make the young doctors better able to contribute to the cooperation between staff and administration so essential to the success of hospitals, wherever they practiced.[40]

During the first four years, while the Duke Hospital was expanding to capacity, all four programs made their primary contributions to the growth of the Duke Hospital staff. In addition to the hospital service which was the core of all four curricula, a large percentage of the graduates of each program stayed on after graduation to take permanent positions at Duke. Once the initial period of expansion ended, however, the graduates began to spread out into other hospitals in the region. Virtually all of the hospital administrators remained in the Carolinas because of the success of The Duke Endowment in placing them in challenging positions.[41] Increasingly, however, Duke was drawing students from outside the region, and in the other three programs this fact was reflected in an increasing dispersion of graduates. At the end of the decade one-third of the graduates of the Duke University School of Nursing were employed by the Duke Hospital, one third lived or practiced elsewhere in North Carolina, and the remainder were dispersed in 19 other states.[42] The Duke Endowment helped to place student dietitians in small hospitals as a part of their training; at the end of the decade graduates were scattered throughout the Carolinas and nine other states.[43] The number of graduates working in assisted hospitals continued to rise but the percentage of graduates so employed declined as more outstanding students, drawn by Duke's increasing national reputation, returned to their home states to practice.

The Duke Endowment required each of its assisted hospitals to file annually, as part of its application for assistance, detailed financial and clinical patient records from each of its departments. The Endowment's central advisory and information service tabulated these records and returned to each hospital a statistical picture of its operations compared to those of other similar hospitals. This picture warned the hospital if it was overspending in any one department or if its professional performance was poor.[44] In the latter cases Rankin frequently consulted members of the Duke medical faculty concerning corrective measures.[45]

The most important single set of consultations concerned Lincoln Hospital in Durham. Aid provided by The Duke Endowment helped to make modern hospital facilities available to Negro physicians in the Carolinas on a scale far beyond the level in other southern states, but the poverty of Negroes generally limited the quality of care which Negro hospitals could offer.[46] Gifts of the Duke family had provided Lincoln with the most modern facilities of any Negro hospital in the region and the Lincoln staff had ready access to the advice of the Duke medical faculty. Yet by 1932, even Lincoln was in trouble. The general health of patients admitted for surgery was so poor that often they had to be fed a balanced diet for a long period just to gain the strength necessary to undergo an operation. Negroes who could afford to pay for their care, and were in correspondingly better health than the indigent, often went to the Duke Hospital. At Lincoln, receipts from patients fell to one-fifth of the annual budget, half the collection rate of other Negro hospitals. Lincoln officials were reluctant to press for payment for fear of losing their remaining patients to Duke.[47] Local doctors admitted to Lincoln's facilities, afraid of losing what little income they received, sometimes attempted surgery beyond their capabilities or before the patient's general condition would permit. When the fatality rate in major operations rose to twice that of the region's other Negro hospitals,[48] the American College of Surgeons withdrew Lincoln's accreditation.

Rankin was determined that Lincoln Hospital should offer a quality of care corresponding to the facilities given by the Duke family and by so doing set a new standard of excellence for medical practice among Negroes. He suggested to Lincoln's trustees that they establish an active consulting staff nominated by the doctors at Duke and Watts Hospitals. These medical consultants would have regular access to Lincoln's facilities, review all cases involving fatality, infectious disease, or complicated treatment with the regular hospital staff, and recommend to the trustees changes in hospital procedures calculated to improve the quality of professional work being done. All this was to be accomplished without removing final responsibility for the hospital from Durham, and particularly its Negro community.[49]

This raised fears among Negro physicians that Duke might absorb Lincoln for teaching purposes and deny them a hospital in which to practice.[50] They argued that to put the institution under white management, and particularly under the partial control of officials of Watts Hospital, where Negroes were not admitted, might strike such a blow at the pride of Durham's Negroes as to cost the hospital its support in the Negro community.[51]

In the face of this sentiment Dean Davison was extremely reluctant to involve Duke Hospital at all in the problem. Without absolute control and complete cooperation, the ill feeling which supervision would cause would only harm the relationship between Duke Hospital and the Negro community without solving Lincoln's problems.[52] The Lincoln trustees, for their part, did not act at all on the proposal until Rankin intimated that The Endowment might withhold its annual contribution. As he saw it, Lincoln had three choices: to let the problem remain; to allow supervision by Duke Hospital; or to allow supervision by the Watts staff.[53]

Unwilling either to risk losing the Endowment's support or to accept supervision by Watts Hospital, the Lincoln trustees turned to Dean Davison for suggestions on how to raise Lincoln's financial and professional service to the standards suggested by The Endowment. His suggestions were even more stringent than Rankin's. He proposed creating an advisory committee to have complete professional and financial responsibility for Lincoln Hospital for five years. The committee, he suggested, should have the endorsement of the Durham City Council and County Commissioners, since both agencies contributed to the hospital's budget. No member of the committee would be allowed to practice at Lincoln. This would remove any suspicion of private gain. He suggested that the committee hire a new business manager to increase collections and a full-time technician to operate the laboratory and x-ray department. He suggested that they appoint a surgical supervisor and a medical supervisor to oversee and approve complicated procedures and a full-time medical resident to supervise the daily work of the hospital. He regarded it as essential that committee members observe the work of the doctors allowed to practice at Lincoln for six months and have complete authority to decide which doctors should continue on the hospital staff. Once the advisory committee chose new staff members for Lincoln it would also supervise their work, particularly by controlling permission for surgery. The logical agency for choosing the advisory committee, Davison said flatly, was the Watts Hospital Board of Trustees.[54]

Durham Negroes could not accept the Davison scheme, for it placed control of a Negro institution entirely in white hands. Lincoln trustee and North Carolina College President James E. Shephard gently reminded Dr. Rankin that part of Washington Duke's purpose in providing the hospital had been to hasten the development of competent Negro leaders. The Lincoln trustees must not be shunted aside, the manager of Lincoln must be a Negro, and the advisory committee must not be controlled entirely by white Watts Hospital.[55] Davison saw in these sentiments only resistance to the concept of outside supervision and repeated his opposition to Duke Hospital participating in the advisory committee.[56]

Despite his opposition, Davison sought the widest possible advice on the situation. Lincoln's problems were not unique, and both he and Rankin hoped that a solution at Lincoln would set a useful precedent for dealing with the problems of Negro hospitals elsewhere in the Carolinas.[57] A possible basis for a solution came from

N. J. Blackwood, medical director of the Provident Hospital in Chicago, whom Davison sounded out on the problem. Control must at first remain entirely with the advisory committee, Blackwood stated, but to be successful it should exercise that control with a gloved hand. This meant implementation by the committee of all of Davison's supervisory proposals. But it also meant referring each decision to the Lincoln trustees for approval.[58] This compromise immediately appealed to Rankin, who believed strongly in the principle of local responsibility.

The Lincoln trustees accepted Davison's suggestion that reorganization of the hospital's financial and professional services be made under the Blackwood formula. An advisory committee of five Durham physicians, including Duke gynecologist Robert A. Ross, received the approval both of the Lincoln trustees and The Duke Endowment, new financial support for Lincoln Hospital from the Julius Rosenwald Foundation, and professional advice from the American College of Surgeons.[59] The committee began the work of reorganization by appointing Negro banker William M. Rich of Norfolk, Virginia as business manager. He revised the financial procedures of the hospital and spent most of his evenings in the churches, lodges, and homes of Durham's Negro community explaining the needs of the hospital and establishing the policy that each patient treated should pay something, however small, toward the cost of his care. The supervising physicians set up an out-patient service and treated most of the charity patients personally. They also organized monthly staff meetings for review of difficult cases, scanned in advance all proposed surgical procedures and participated in the operations actually conducted. They also cleared from the hospital all persons with chronic illnesses which could be effectively treated at home.[60]

The completeness of the takeover reawakened fears among Negro physicians that they would not be allowed to resume their full practice even after the period of observation. Here personal diplomacy proved decisive. Durham physician N. O. Spikes, chairman of the advisory committee, adamantly insisted on giving Negro physicians every opportunity to qualify for staff privileges. His dedication won the support of North Carolina Mutual Insurance Company president, C. C. Spaulding, chairman of the hospital's finance committee.

Spaulding's influence insured that Durham Negroes would give the experiment a fair trial.[61]

Within months the benefits of supervision became obvious. The mortality rate among patients dropped back toward expected limits, and the percentage of care given on a charity basis dropped as collections improved. From the improved collections funds were set aside to be matched by grants from The Duke Endowment to purchase a new heating plant and badly needed equipment.[62] Business manager Rich, working with the Hospital Care Association, worked out an insurance program for Negroes which provided up to 25 days of hospitalization per year at an annual cost of $4.24 as part of his effort to help Lincoln's patients pay more toward the cost of their care. As conditions in the hospital improved and as more Negro physicians qualified for staff privileges, the last vestiges of resentment over supervision disappeared. Duke and Lincoln doctors cooperated in presenting a clinic on diseases of the chest at Lincoln, modeled on the Duke Medical School symposia, open to all Negro physicians in the Carolinas and Virginia.[63] At the end of two years the Lincoln trustees and staff once again were in complete control of their hospital,[64] which was becoming the model Negro hospital Rankin had envisioned.

Dean Davison's role in designing a mechanism for reorganizing Lincoln Hospital was the most important example of how the Duke medical faculty helped to solve problems in assisted hospitals revealed by the statistical analyses compiled by The Duke Endowment. Davison's work helped Lincoln regain accreditation by the American College of Surgeons. The Duke University School of Medicine also helped assisted hospitals to maintain standards of medical practice warranting certification by national accrediting agencies. The American College of Surgeons required that doctors in approved hospitals submit all tissues removed during operations to clinical pathological laboratories to get aid in diagnosing difficult cases and to review the necessity and effectiveness of all surgical procedures.[65] Rural communities, however, could afford neither to build such laboratories nor to employ on a full-time basis one of the few trained pathologists in North Carolina.

Officials of local hospitals were similarly concerned to meet these standards, and some approached the Duke professor of pathology,

Dr. Wiley Forbus, about doing the laboratory work for their hospitals.[66] In consultation with Rankin, Forbus developed a plan for an outside pathological service for institutions assisted by The Duke Endowment.[67] Participating hospitals would be invited to send all pathological material removed at operation or obtained at autopsy for examination at Duke.[68] In addition to sending reports of each case to the local hospital involved, the Duke pathology department would keep permanent records of all cases for comparative study and invited physicians from the local hospitals to come to Duke for postgraduate education based upon their own case material.[69] Dr. Forbus proposed to charge a low flat rate of $25 per month for this service, regardless of the number of cases submitted, in order to interest small hospitals in the program.[70] He estimated that the participation of 25 hospitals would enable him to hire staff sufficient to process all incoming specimens without lowering the quality of work done by the Duke department.

Rankin anticipated little trouble in finding 25 customer hospitals.[71] So great was the need for diagnostic pathology service that the cases sent in for report by the first fifteen subscribing institutions exceeded in number those done for Duke Hospital. Not enough hospitals enrolled, however, to make the program self-supporting. With his staff limited by the University budget, Forbus feared that the quantity of work would compromise the quality of the examinations his department performed.[72] Since the cost of processing each case exceeded two dollars and the participating hospitals were sending more than 13 cases monthly, Duke Hospital absorbed much of the cost of work done for the smaller institutions.[73] Only a grant from The Duke Endowment underwriting the operating deficits of the first two years allowed Forbus to continue.

The failure of the staffs of many small hospitals to subscribe to the plan was caused in some cases by limited budgets, but more often by opposition to the idea of an outside agency reviewing their practice for errors. Rural medicine was not practiced under ideal conditions. Patients traveled long distances to reach what hospitals there were. When a patient presented a clinical impression which might require a minor operation, such as an appendectomy, doctors often preferred to perform the surgery without complete diagnostic study rather than risk having the patient return home and suffer complications while unable to reach a hospital. Forbus considered the most important single service he could perform for the small hospitals to be a review of proposed and accomplished surgery which would help to eliminate unnecessary operations.[74] Some of his first customers, however, protested receiving reports on removed appendixes marked "normal organ," and at least one accused Forbus of incompetence.[75]

When complaints arose, Forbus's collected library of specimens became a valuable rejoinder and teaching device. He asked offended physicians to come to Duke and review the specimens and the reports in the laboratory. Forbus's notations in the margins of letters of complaint indicate that this procedure allowed him to settle disputes to the satisfaction of all involved.[76]

As Forbus's reports aided more and more physicians to plan surgery and make complicated diagnoses more accurately, the climate of opinion changed and enough hospitals began to subscribe to make the pathology service self-supporting. The Duke Medical School benefitted along with the participating hospitals. The larger staff made possible by income from the service also made possible more effective teaching of pathology to smaller groups of medical students. At the same time, the clinical material sent in by the participating hospitals made it possible for Dr. Forbus to train more of his instructors as graduate clinical pathologists.[77] The service also strengthened the position of Duke Hospital as the referral center for the state. It encouraged the small hospitals to send clinically interesting patients and patients important to Duke's research projects as well as specimens to Duke for examination.[78]

Neither Forbus nor The Duke Endowment, however, saw the service as a means of supporting the department of pathology. The goal of the service was to upgrade and support standards of medical practice in areas where the members of the local medical profession had not the training or resources to do the laboratory work themselves. Whenever a hospital was able to obtain the services of a trained pathologist in its own locality, Forbus encouraged it to do so.[79] As more pathologists settled in North Carolina, they helped to keep the growth of Forbus's service within the limits of its position as a part of a teaching department. The number of participating hospitals fluctuated between 25 and 30 throughout the decade, new institutions replacing those which became able, with the assistance of The Duke Endowment, to perform or obtain pathological diagnostic service locally.[80]

With the average age of physicians in rural areas increasing and their skills increasingly dated,[81] the effective use of hospitals depended in part upon providing country doctors with opportunities for postgraduate education. Fewer than one each year, however, accepted Davison's standing invitation to the profession of the Carolinas and Virginia to attend classes or study in the laboratories at Duke,[82] nor was Forbus's cumulative file often used by local doctors except in cases of disagreement. Apparently many doctors, like most citizens, were "not educated to hospital mindedness."[83]

The alternative to extensive study by individuals was intensive study by groups, the approach developed in the Duke University medical symposia. In the fall of each year, beginning in 1934, every doctor in the Carolinas and Virginia was invited to attend an annual weekend series of lectures and demonstrations by national medical authorities at the Duke Hospital. Each symposium attempted to make a comprehensive presentation of recent developments in the symposium subject area.[84] Each year a new specialty was featured. A local doctor might choose to attend only one of the annual programs, but if he came every year he would within five years have updated his skills in each major division of medical practice: surgery, medicine, pediatrics, obstetrics and gynecology. He could meet not only his friends but also national medical authorities, both in the classroom and at the Duke football game which always closed the weekend.[85]

The first symposium attracted almost 300 persons, and their response was overwhelmingly favorable. The next year the attendance doubled.[86] At each symposium emphasis was placed primarily upon the difficulty of accurate diagnosis and upon the value of the laboratory facilities of local hospitals as aids to the general practitioner.[87] Demonstrations showing new discoveries and techniques were set up and staffed by Duke faculty and kept open after the formal close of the symposium so that each doctor could have all his questions answered.[88]

Even those doctors who resented the professional competition of the Duke faculty recognized the value of the program and applauded its appearance. Rankin saw the symposium not only as a means of upgrading the medical practice in the region but also as "the most powerful answer and the most embarrassing answer" to medical critics of the work of The Duke Endowment and the Duke University Medical School.[89] The programs attracted not only doctors, but also nurses, administrators, and leading citizens interested in medicine. By the end of the decade attendance at some sessions exceeded 1000 persons.[90]

As the size of the crowds increased, however, the goal of providing a comprehensive review of a specialty area for each person attending became increasingly unwieldy. This goal presupposed that all the doctors would be able to attend every important lecture, clinic, or demonstration given during the weekend. The complete postgraduate course in gastrointestinal diseases offered 17 major lectures and clinics in a single day running from 9:00 A.M. to midnight and broken only for meals and occasional ten-minute intermissions.[91] Even physicians accustomed to long hours of work found this schedule strenuous.

Gradually the pedagogy of the symposia changed. Although the attempt still was made each year to cover major topics and new developments within a specialty area, the idea of providing comprehensive review was dropped. Presentations became fewer in number, and question periods longer. Increasingly evening meetings were given over to round-table discussions and banquets, at which the local doctors more easily met the symposia faculty individually or in small groups and listened not only to their knowledge of medical practice but also to their attitude about it.[92] Davison's own attitudes toward the practice of medicine were substantially shaped by his encounters with "great" doctors. Now Duke offered the physicians of the area brief but similar opportunities.

The symposium format also was used to deal with statewide health care problems. Forbus used it in 1933 to bring together at Duke pathologists from throughout the South to exchange ideas on how best to teach pathology in the medical schools and to provide the region with widely dispersed laboratory pathologists.[93] In 1939 the Duke Hospital and The Duke Endowment offered a two-week refresher course for hospital administrators throughout the region to acquaint them with new techniques in nursing education, keeping medical records, administering group hospitalization plans, and recruiting physicians for rural areas.[94] Clinics similar to those offered at Duke were provided at Lincoln Hospital for Negro physicians in the Carolinas and Virginia beginning in 1936.[95] In 1940, Lincoln hosted the first of a series of annual tri-state refresher courses for administrators, bookkeepers, and record librarians of Negro hospitals.[96] These and similar symposia in other fields not only brought new information to bear on medical care problems but also fostered the personal relationships necessary, in the absence of governmental participation, for comprehensive health planning on statewide and regional levels.

By the end of the thirties The Duke Endowment was spending one million dollars annually to support the operation of 129 hospitals in the Carolinas.[97] Rankin considered it "very likely" that the central advisory and information services of The Endowment enabled these hospitals to save as much as they were given, or another 15 percent of their total operating costs.[98] Between 1924 and 1939, using its funds as leverage to extract appropriations from local governments, The Endowment helped to build, equip, or purchase 73 hospitals for local communities. Of the total cost of these projects The Endowment contributed only 38 percent. The number of general hospital beds available in the Carolinas rose from 5431 to 10,057, an increase of 85 percent. Relative to population beds increased from 1.2 per thousand to 1.8 per thousand, or 50 percent. Only 12 percent of the general hospital beds in the Carolinas were in private proprietary hospitals, compared to 51 percent when The Duke Endowment began its work.[99] These improvements were the direct result of the Endowment's support for hospital operations and construction and its central hospital advisory service.

The number of patients using hospitals increased almost twice as fast as the number of beds available. In 1924 the general hospitals of the Carolinas treated 100,669 patients, in 1939, 256,883, an increase of 155 percent. This influx was successfully accommodated in part because improvements in the quality of professional care reduced the average period of treatment of patients in general hospitals from 10.7 to 9.3 days, a decrease of 13 percent.[100]

To this improvement the Duke University School of Medicine and Hospital made significant contributions. To the new public hospitals, staffed increasingly by Duke nurses, technicians, and administrators, came more and more young physicians. The south-eastern United States had fewer physicians in 1940 than in 1927 despite a rise in population. In the Carolinas, however, the reverse was true. North Carolina led the entire region with an increase of 18 percent.[101] Two of every three Carolinians graduated from Duke remained in the state to practice. More important, one of every six graduates and one of every four interns or residents born out of state remained in the Carolinas.[102] The Duke medical faculty contributed even more directly to the quality of health care in the Carolinas by advising hospitals with serious problems when these were revealed by the statistics compiled by The Duke Endowment, aiding many hospitals to review the quality of their professional care through the outside pathological service, assisting in different diagnostic cases through the mechanism of the Duke out-patient clinics, and providing general practitioners with opportunities to retool through the Duke medical symposia.

The success of these experiments in privately financed comprehensive planning for modern health care on a statewide basis while retaining the principle of local control over health facilities, apportioning funds according to need wherever local communities were willing to pay part of the cost, was unique in America. One result of the depression was to reverse completely the roles of government and private funds in the development of hospitals. By 1937 the federal government was paying over three-fourths of the total cost of hospital construction in the United States, largely through its P.W.A. and W.P.A. programs (see Table 4). Much of this federal

Table 4. Capital investment of governmental and nongovernmental funds in hospitals, 1927–37

| | Investment and percentage distribution | | |
	1927	1932	1937
Government	$ 38,505,605 (28.5)	$ 18,156,080 (79.5)	$70,387,392 (71.5)
Nongovernment	95,845,000 (71.5)	5,732,635 (20.5)	28,674,600 (28.5)
Total	134,350,605 (100)	23,888,715 (100)	99,061,992 (100)

Note—Table taken from Michael M. Davis, "Who Finances Construction?" in Arthur C. Bachmeyer, ed., *The Hospital In Modern Society*, p. 62.

investment was concentrated in those few populous states able to meet P.W.A. matching fund requirements.[103]

Franklin Delano Roosevelt considered the health needs of the nation a matter of social security.[104] Under this heading the greater medical needs of rural areas and less wealthy states could not be ignored. Roosevelt appointed an Interdepartmental Committee for Coordination of Federal Health Services in 1935 to survey the nation's health needs.[105] In 1937 Surgeon General Thomas H. Parran asked Rankin for an opportunity to tour the community hospitals of the Carolinas assisted by The Endowment to study their effect in drawing young physicians to rural areas and in upgrading the level of medical practice. A similar study was made the next year by Dr. Vane M. Hoge of the U. S. Public Health Service.[106]

In February, 1938, the committee reported to Roosevelt that although the total numbers of physicians and hospital beds in the country were approximately sufficient to meet demands for service, at least one-third and perhaps one-half of the population lived in medical poverty either because of limited income or because no hospital facilities existed in sparsely settled areas. To meet these needs the committee recommended, in addition to increasing available public health services created by the Social Security Act, the construction of some 500 to 600 hospitals of 50 to 60 beds to provide medical care in and attract physicians to rural areas. In addition the committee urged some form of insurance or tax support to enable families of moderate income to minimize the financial burdens of unexpected illness, and increased government financial support for services furnished to persons without income.[107] The model system of health care and delivery now proposed for the nation, in short, was exactly that undertaken for the Carolinas by The Duke Endowment in cooperation with the Duke University School of Medicine and Hospital.

Eight years passed before the Hill-Burton Act gave the federal government by law the primary responsibility for expansion of the nation's health care facilities which the depression gave it in fact. During those years the collective experience of The Duke Endowment, Duke Hospital, and the Duke University School of Medicine in helping the people of the Carolinas to take financial responsibility for their health care needs remained the best evidence for the administration's contention that local communities could successfully assume financial responsibility for federally constructed hospitals.[108] The Duke experience was one of the resources available to the Senate Committee on Education and Labor during the hearings on the Hill-Burton bill.[109] Senator Allen Ellender of Louisiana indirectly applauded the pioneer work of the institutions created by James B. Duke in the area of comprehensive medical care by observing to one North Carolina witness before the committee, "it is not every State that is fortunate enough to have a Duke in its midst, you know."[110] In the final bill the principles of comprehensive planning for health care on a statewide basis, local control of plans and facilities, provision of beds for the indigent in each hospital constructed, apportioning of funds according to need and, in the first drafts, requiring states to match federal funds according to their relative wealth directly reflected the principles of The Duke Endowment in dealing with the communities of the Carolinas.

Chapter 9: The Regional Medical Center: End of an Era, 1940–1941

The creation of a Department of Neuropsychiatry and the construction of a hospital wing to house the Private Diagnostic Clinics mark the division between two eras of Duke University medicine. By contributing a percentage of their earnings from private practice to a development fund in lieu of rent on the new clinical facilities, the medical faculty began to take over from the University both initiative and financial responsibility for the future expansion of the plant as well as the program of the medical school and hospital. The new wing, with two floors of offices and examining rooms for the Medical and Surgical Private Diagnostic Clinics, and 113 additional private and semiprivate beds, enlarged the space available for each physician's private practice enough to foresee the financing of future expansion of facilities largely out of funds accumulated by assessing each doctor a small percentage of his gross earnings.

The completion of the new wing freed the former house staff dormitory on the third floor of the hospital for conversion into a ward for psychiatric patients.[1] Neuropsychiatry was the last of the originally envisioned departments of the medical school to be funded. During the first decade neuropsychiatry was taught as a function of the department of medicine, briefly by Ernest M. Poate and, from 1933, by Raymond G. Crispell, former student of Adolph Meyer at The Johns Hopkins. Crispell's teaching, founded on Meyer's conceptualizations, had a practical common sense quality. Eleven clinics introduced second-year students to psychobiology and psychopathology, and in addition students were required to apply their new knowledge by examining the makeup of their own personalities for purposes of better self-understanding. Junior students heard lectures relating psychiatric concepts to neurology and internal medicine. Seniors attended clinics at Duke showing psychiatric problems common on hospital wards and outpatient services and at state institutions dealing with more severe cases.[2] Although Crispell carried a patient load of 600 to 660 per year,[3] there were no facilities at Duke for primary psychiatric cases, a situation which left no opportunity for students to learn to work, under supervision, with major psychiatric problems.

The State of North Carolina was similarly short of psychiatric care facilities. This situation prompted Dean Davison, Dr. Hanes, and Dr. Crispell to draft a resolution, approved by the state legislature, calling for a survey of mental health needs in North Carolina. They then secured supporting funds from the Rockefeller Foundation for the proposed study. In its final report, the study commission concluded that it was "humanly impossible" for the patients in state mental hospitals to obtain proper care and attention. In the state institutions low per capita costs were counted the primary mark of effectiveness and the ratio of physicians to patients was currently one to 528, as against the standard of one to 150 recommended by the American Psychiatric Association. Among the recommendations included in the report was one urging Duke to establish a full department of psychiatry, a psychiatric hospital of at least 50 beds, and an out-patient clinic to train specialists for private practice and mental hospitals throughout the state.[4]

In his letter transmitting the study to Governor J. C. B. Ehringhaus, Dr. Hanes warned that it was "too often the fate of official reports to find themselves quietly interred in the oblivion of dusty pidgeon-holes."[5] Despite the warning, this was exactly what happened.[6]

When it became clear that the State would do nothing to implement the Commission's report, Davison approached Dr. Alan Gregg of the Rockefeller Foundation for funds to develop a department of psychiatry at Duke and thereby realize, at least in part, the objectives of the Foundation in underwriting the original study of mental health care in North Carolina.[7] While this proposal was under consideration Dr. Robert S. Carroll, longtime proprietor of a private mental hospital in Asheville, North Carolina, offered his hospital as an outright gift to Duke University.[8] The acceptance of this gift and the projected opening of the new psychiatric ward in the Duke Hospital itself moved the Rockefeller Foundation to approve a grant of $175,000 over seven years to support a full department of neuropsychiatry.[9] Dr. Richard S. Lyman of The Johns Hopkins was appointed professor to head the new department. His coming, the gift of Highland Hospital, and the new private clinic wing completed the original design of the Duke University Medical School and Hospital.

The completion of the original dream for the Duke University School of Medicine and Hospital with the opening of the psychiatric facilities affords an opportunity to consider the accomplishment in some perspective. Four factors beyond all others manifestly shaped the new institution. The first was the medical poverty of the rural South. History committed Duke University to the attempt to stop the continuing migration of patients, medical sudents, and doctors from the region in search of competent treatment, clinical training, and more rewarding opportunities to practice. The second was the standard of medical education set by The Johns Hopkins University School of Medicine and confirmed by the Flexner report in 1910, based on laboratory science in the preclinical years, bedside teaching as the medium for teaching the art of medicine, and close personal contact between the students and their professors. Many of the members of the pioneer generation at Duke came directly, or almost directly, from their Hopkins experience (see appendix 3). Third was the size of the bequests of James B. Duke, which guaranteed the new institution the finest facilities in the South and the opportunity of cooperating with The Duke Endowment in the attempt to modernize medicine in the Carolinas. Finally, the depression, which forced the members of the medical faculty to be efficient as clinicians and innovative as administrators.

These four factors standing alone would never have produced the successful institution that evolved had it not been for the vision, historical imagination, and the willpower of the dean, Dr. Wilburt C. Davison, who mobilized the resources to deal with the environment in which the new school arose.[10] His success was the product of a willingness to gamble in appointing a young, Hopkins-trained faculty and the ability to build out of his personal experience a practical set of priorities for developing the medical school and hospital and a compatible strategy for modernizing medicine in the Carolinas.

The gamble on a young, relatively unknown faculty was born in part of necessity—the new school could not pay salaries large enough to attract full professors from established institutions. But Davison's tactic was born primarily of knowledge. The Hopkins itself was first developed by young doctors. The medical training given at The Hopkins was superior to that offered elsewhere because of the close relation between laboratory and bedside instruction, the opportunity to observe the "great doctors" on the faculty at close hand, and the unequaled traffic of guest medical specialists through the lecture halls, clinics, and conventions in Baltimore. Many southerners studying at The Hopkins wished for a promising opportunity to contribute to improving the practice of medicine in their native region. Men trained together in a successful institution and tradition seemed more likely to work together well in a new situation. What Davison's first faculty lacked in broad experience it gained back in zeal, familiarity with a common pattern of operation, and unity in the conviction that Duke's primary objective must be to provide a basic, practical education for its students, expressed first and foremost in the ability to make accurate clinical diagnoses.

Davison described his deanship in terms that reflected his wartime experience. He called himself the adjutant of the faculty, not the commanding officer. This terminology allowed him freedom in two directions. As adjutant he alone was party to all of the discussions of the medical school faculty, the administrative conference, university officials, and the Duke Endowment staff. Sitting at the hub of medical activities at Duke, only he could see both needs and possibilities throughout the organization as a whole and allocate funds accordingly. During the depression, with each professor absorbed in making his new department succeed and seeing only his own sector of activity, fiscal leverage afforded Davison a position of absolute power. But in styling himself as adjutant rather than commander the appearance of his authority was minimized. As adjutant he was free to exploit his genuinely informal personal style, always available to anyone and everyone, able to disagree without bitterness, quick to emphasize the partnership of administration, staff and students in building the new institution.

Davison's availability set the style both for administration and teaching at Duke. Both began with delegation of full authority for the task at hand and freedom to experiment in its accomplishment. Each person, at whatever task, was expected to seek help when he needed it and to succeed in the end; and everyone, faculty and students alike, soon came to understand this pervasive spirit of cooperation. Participation in achievement built confidence in individuals and individual commitment to the institution.

Given the needs of the area, limited financial resources, and the faculty's philosophy which stressed diagnostic ability above all else, it is not surprising that the public and private diagnostic clinics were the unique contribution of Duke to medicine during the first decade. The first need of the medical school was for an adequate number and variety of patients. The first need of the people of the Carolinas was for a hospital offering specialty care at reasonable cost. Before Duke opened its doors the practice of medicine in North Carolina had been decentralized, a cottage industry. Patients requiring complicated procedures went North, to Philadelphia or Baltimore, if they could pay; often they received no treatment if they could not. Now by the tens of thousands they came to Duke, traveling an average of 70 miles to avail themselves of group diagnostic service. Now it was possible for general practitioners to obtain help with their diagnostic problems in both pay and charity cases, thereby strengthening their local practices. During the first ten years over 150,000 patients made more than half a million visits to the Duke Hospital.[11] Duke was the referral hospital, and Durham the medical center, of the region.

Experimentation with distributing the cost of medical care more evenly across the population logically followed from the clinic concept. The clinics themselves reduced the cost to the patient of the services of each physician by minimizing the time each physician spent per case and reducing the hospital space required to accommodate large numbers of patients. The flat rate plan spread the cost of hospital services more evenly across the patient population. The cooperative plan, based on the principle that each patient should pay something for medical care according to his means, sought systematically to enlist the voluntary support of families, friends, charitable organizations, and government agencies so that by reducing the charity burden on the hospital in any single case, care could be offered to a greater number of persons. By the end of the decade hospitalization insurance allowed over 200,000 North Carolinians of moderate means to budget for their hospital care.

Teaching and research alike were grounded in the service given by the hospital. The preclinical students learned in the laboratory to identify the structures and functions of the human body, to recognize the effects of disease, and to perform the tests necessary to isolate and evaluate clinical problems. The students in their clinical years, the interns, and the residents, mastered the art of medicine by moving through staged levels of responsibility for patient care on the wards and in the out-patient clinics, which screened the patients for admission to the wards. The faculty's research activity grew almost entirely out of the clinical problems encountered among patients and out of tests made on new therapeutic procedures developed to meet them.

In partnership with The Duke Endowment, the Medical School and Hospital helped to improve medical care throughout the Carolinas. Duke doctors, nurses, technicians, and administrators increasingly manned the general hospitals constructed throughout the region, many built or equipped through the leverage of Duke Endowment grants. The standards of practice in these same hospitals were raised by the operational analyses furnished by The Endowment, the consulting services of Duke's medical faculty, the surgical supervision of the outside pathological service, and the retraining of local doctors through the Duke symposia.

The progress of Duke's first decade came in meeting the problems of the regional medical environment. The clinics, the curriculum, the rate structures, the insurance plans, the research projects, the services to other hospitals, all were designed to meet the local shortages of physicians, facilities, and dollars. Together they formed a strategy of modernization of health services based on the principles of centralized diagnostic service and care for the critically ill, multiplication of local doctors' skills through the provision of hospitals and supporting personnel, and generalization of the costs of medical care, through voluntary cooperation wherever possible. Taken together they reversed the decline in the availability of up-to-date health care in the Carolinas and built the clinical patronage necessary for a teaching hospital.

The environment resisted every advance. The complex of institutions created by James B. Duke reversed in the Carolinas the decline in the availability of medical care common elsewhere in the South during the depression decade. Those institutions by themselves, however, could not greatly improve the level of medical care available compared to states outside the region. North Carolina remained within the bottom quarter of the states with respect to the ratio of doctors to population, the ratio of hospital beds to population, net income per capita, and average educational level of adults in the population.[12] Poverty and rural isolation continued to deprive many patients of care, even at low cost. The widely scattered farm population was not easily enrolled in or encouraged to budget for hospital insurance. Moreover, rural students rarely possessed the combination of means and premedical training needed to attend medical school. Because the Duke Medical School was limited, for teaching effectiveness, to 76 students per class and committed to accepting none but the best possible students, Duke could do little more to supply the region with doctors unless the quality of rural applicants improved.

Gradually state officials adopted the Duke model as a political objective under the slogan "More Doctors, More Hospitals, More Insurance."[13] The first promise of substantial help in meeting the region's medical problems, however, came out of a replay of the cooperative medical school controversy of the 1920's. At the urging of the medical profession, the 1937 North Carolina General Assembly authorized Governor Clyde R. Hoey to appoint a commission to investigate the state's need for another four-year medical school and report back to the 1939 Assembly. Either the University of North Carolina or the Wake Forest College school could be expanded, or the two could be joined.[14] Davison supported the general purpose of the commission, believing that there was sufficient place in North Carolina for another four-year school.[15] The deans of both the two-year schools were members of the commission.

During the commission's deliberations Mr. Odus M. Mull, State Representative from Shelby and also a commission member, reported that a committee to select the beneficiary of a large charitable bequest was interested in making a commitment to the proposed new medical school if it could be located in the donor's home city, Winston-Salem. A majority of the commission, however, would not consider any location other than Chapel Hill for the four-year school and 300 bed hospital which they recommended be added to the University of North Carolina. The state, unfortunately, lacked funds for the project, so the recommendation died.[16]

Immediately after the commission filed its report, Dean Coy C. Carpenter of the Wake Forest School asked Mull to inquire of the family of Bowman Gray, the source of the bequest, whether they

would commit his legacy to the expansion of the Wake Forest College school if it moved to Winston-Salem and united with the North
Carolina Baptist Hospital.[17] The faculty of the Wake Forest school
had desired for more than a decade to combine all services for care
of the sick sponsored by North Carolina Baptists in one place.[18] In
1935 the American Medical Association's Council on Medical Education voted not to accredit further any two-year schools. This decision
was reversed when the Association of American Medical Colleges
protested,[19] an action in which Davison played a leading role,[20] but it
confirmed Wake Forest's desire to expand.[21] With the gift of the
Bowman Gray Fund, 18,500 shares of R. J. Reynolds Tobacco Company "B" common stock valued at approximately $600,000, that
dream was realized.[22]

The Bowman Gray School of Medicine opened in 1941 in a
wing of the North Carolina Baptist Hospital built with a loan secured by the tobacco stock. At the laying of the cornerstone Duke's
Dean Davison pointed out that soon North Carolina would benefit
from having two medical centers. The state would have to depend
less on physicians migrating in from other areas as the new school
trained more doctors. Its people would have two teaching institutions with diagnostic clinics to serve them, and its physicians new
possibilities for postgraduate training.[23] With a second four-year
medical school open in the state and supporters of the state university
promoting still a third, Duke anticipated sharing its regional responsibilities and developing its national reputation as a teaching and
research center.

The shadow of war, however, clouded the future. As late as April,
1940, Duke refused invitations by the Army and Navy to form medical units for overseas service in national emergencies because of
heavy patient and teaching loads. Then the invasion of France made
it increasingly probable that the United States would be involved in
the war. When Duke's acceptance of an invitation to form a Navy
unit was not acted upon for three months, the medical faculty informed Major General James C. Magee, the Surgeon General of the
Army, of its willingness to form a General Hospital unit similar to
North Carolina Base Hospital No. 65 of the First World War, which
Hanes had commanded. On October 17, 1940, the Surgeon General
accepted the proposal.[24]

Davison learned the probable consequences of war for Duke at a conference with officials at the War Department. Present and former members of the teaching and house staff and Duke alumni elsewhere with at least one year of internship experience were eligible for commissions in the new 65th General Hospital. From these groups the 66 medical officers for the new unit, designed to care for up to 1000 patients,[25] would be chosen. All interns, residents, and other physicians under 36 years of age holding reserve commissions, he was told, could expect to be called to active service within six months, with those still in hospital training likely to be called first unless considered by local draft boards to be essential for hospital or other needs. Medical students lacking one year of internship experience could probably expect deferment, but Davison advised them to obtain Medical Reserve commissions and to request active service at the completion of their first year of internship without being drafted, in view of the Army's need for doctors. Heads of departments were authorized to defer appointments to assistant residencies and residencies at Duke Hospital until the completion of a student's active service. As a matter of policy, Duke granted intern credit to Duke graduates drafted after one year of internship for active service. Davison hoped, however, that these men would return to hospitals for further internships or residencies upon discharge.[26]

Dr. Elbert L. Persons, Jr., assistant professor of medicine, was appointed unit director of the 65th and chief of the medical service. Dr. Clarence E. Gardner, Jr., professor of surgery, became chief of the surgical service and Julia E. White, Assistant to the Dean of the School of Nursing, the unit's chief nurse. These three were primarily responsible for recruiting the staff of the 65th.[27]

While Persons, Gardner, and Miss White organized the staff of the hospital unit, Davison, aided by Forbus and Swett, laid plans for continuing to operate the Duke medical school and hospital with only those doctors who were absolutely essential to teaching and patient care.[28] Medical students also had to be classified as to availability for service. The armed forces required their medical officers to have both a degree and a year of internship experience. Since the medical schools graduated annually fewer doctors than the military needed, the schools sought Class II-A deferment of their students, until completion of one year of postgraduate training, as men necessary to the national health.[29] Selective Service directives recognized the dangerously low level of manpower in the medical profession, but by law authority to grant deferments rested with local boards in each individual case.[30] Some local boards did not consider hospital internship justification for II-A classification,[31] so Davison spent long hours trying to compose a letter of request for deferment that would favorably influence local board members.[32]

The war news increasingly dominated the University atmosphere. "It is a time," said Hanes at the November dedication of the Department of Neuropsychiatry, "to shake man's faith in man, but it is also a very fitting time to dedicate to the service of sick mankind one more small evidence that medicine holds fast to sanity in a world that seems violently insane."[33] In the months that followed, some 200 faculty, including most of the senior professors in the medical school, organized themselves informally as the Duke Council for American Defense in order to survey the resources of the University useful in a national emergency and generally to inform the local community and prepare it for whatever turn the war might take.[34]

By October, 1941, the future seemed clear. The annual symposium, on the topic "Problems of Civil and Military Emergencies," featured several specialists just returned from the bombed cities of Britain.[35] The headlines of the morning papers reported the advance of German armies toward Moscow, the fall of the third Ronoye government in Japan, and the first successful torpedo attack against a U.S. warship.[36] For the staff of the 65th General Hospital the symposium was a training obligation.[37] The number of Duke graduates and former house staff members called to the colors was rising rapidly— 84 would be on active service before Pearl Harbor.[38] Davison's Princeton classmate and fellow Rhodes scholar, Wilder G. Penfield of the Montreal Neurological Institute, set the tone of the symposium in a paper pointing up the surprising absence of mental disorders in war-torn Britain. Bombings and privations, he noted, far from breaking British morale, "strengthened the Britishers' nerves and crystalized their determination to see this dreadful war through."[39] No one who heard him doubted that they must soon do likewise.

Appendices

Appendix 1. Statistics of the Duke University Schools of Medicine, Nursing, and Dietetics, and Duke Hospital, 1930–1940

	1930–31	1931–32	1932–33	1933–34	1934–35	1935–36	1936–37	1937–38	1938–39	1939–40	Totals
Medical students	70	144	165	193	210	217	241	244	256	259	696[a]
Medical graduates[b]	0	17(5)	14(3)	34(5)	48(8)	38(12)	54(6)	51(11)	60	58(5)	374(55)
Interns and residents	16	33	41	49	57	64	71	80	85	86	312[c]
Pupil nurses	33	60	74	69	69	65	78	82	98	119	402[d]
Nursing graduates[e]			14	22	19	15(1)	19(6)	18(19)	23(18)	21(19)	151(63)
Student dietitians	1	3	3	4	4	4	4	4	6	6	39
Total patients[f]	6,248	15,754	26,422	39,796	54,659	69,469	87,095	104,136	122,810	143,180	143,180[g]
Average daily patient census	91	143	193	234	279	308	311	316	350	375	
Maximum daily census				278	339	348	355	360	389	433	
Total days of hospital care	42,269	60,362	69,521	78,103	92,336	109,150	113,654	115,474	127,710	137,307	945,886
Percentage of part and full charity	62	65	79	76	66	68	64	56	56	52	
Total visits in public dispensary	9,581	22,959	24,428	32,938	37,641	38,026	49,538	52,364	66,946	85,536	419,957
Scientific publications by staff and students	33	38	41	45	56	62	87	124	126	204	816

a. 627 first-year, 5 second-year, and 64 junior students (total 696) were admitted 1930–39 inclusive from 6,986 applicants.
b. The first figure indicates those who received the degree of Doctor of Medicine and that in parentheses those who also received the degree of Bachelor of Science in Medicine.
c. Total interns, assistant residents, and residents who have spent 1–7 years in Duke Hospital, 1930–39.
d. Total first-year pupil nurses admitted 1930–39.
e. The first figure indicates those who received the Diploma in Nursing and that in parentheses those who also received the degree of Bachelor of Science in Nursing.
f. These figures are cumulative; each new patient (Hospital, Public Dispensary and Private Diagnostic Clinics) is given a consecutive number which remains the same regardless of the number of times he or she returns to the Hospital.
g. On July 21, 1940, the tenth anniversary of the opening of the Hospital, the 144,142nd patient was registered.
Note—This table is taken by permission of the editor of the *North Carolina Medical Journal* from Wilburt C. Davison, "The First Ten Years of Duke University School of Medicine and Duke Hospital," *North Carolina Medical Journal* 2 (Oct. 1941): 529.

Appendix 2. Additional hospital statistics, 1930–1941

	Number of beds	Occupancy rate	Average stay (in days)	Cost per bed day
1930	156	58.2%	14.7	$11.17
1931	284	50.7	12.9	7.28
1932	339	54.5	12.0	5.66
1933	338	59.3	12.1	4.61
1934	375	62.9	10.6	4.69
1935	388	71.3	11.5	4.90
1936	414	74.6	10.5	4.58
1937	416	73.6	10.2	5.15
1938	418	83.9	11.2	5.49
1939	425	88.1	11.5	5.49
1940	498	86.4	11.4	5.57
1941	498	78.6	11.9	5.79

Appendix 3. Original Faculty of the Schools of Medicine, Nursing and Health Services, 1930–1931[1]

Name	Title
Frederick Vernon Altvater	Intern in Hospital Administration
*Edwin Pascal Alyea, S.B., M.D.	Instructor in Urology
*Harold Lindsay Amoss, S.B., M.S., Dr.B.H., Sc.D., M.D.	Professor of Medicine
*William Banks Anderson, A.B., M.D.	Instructor in Otolaryngology
*Bessie Baker, B.S., R.N.	Dean of School of Nursing and Professor of Nursing Education
*Roger Denio Baker, A.B., M.D.	Instructor in Anatomy
*Frederick Bernheim, A.B., Ph.D.	Assistant Professor of Physiology
*Mary Lilias Christian Bernheim, B.A., M.A., Ph.D.	Instructor in Biochemistry
*Bayard Carter, A.B., B.A., M.A., M.D.	Professor of Obstetrics and Gynecology
*Wilburt Cornell Davison, A.B., B.A., B.Sc., M.A., M.D., D.Sc., LL.D.	Dean of School of Medicine and Professor of Pediatrics
*George Sharpe Eadie, B.A., M.A., M.B., Ph.D.	Professor of Physiology and Pharmacology
*Watt Weems Eagle, A.B., M.D.	Assistant Professor of Otolaryngology
Judith Farrar, A.B., B.S.	Medical Librarian
Mildred Perkins Farrar, A.B.	Assistant Medical Librarian
*Wiley Davis Forbus, A.B., M.D.	Professor of Pathology
*Clarence Ellsworth Gardner, Jr., A.B., M.D.	Resident in Surgery
Edwin Crowell Hamblen, B.S., M.D.	Associate Professor of Obstetrics and Gynecology
*Frederic Moir Hanes, A.B., A.M., M.D.	Associate Professor of Medicine
*Oscar Carl Edward Hansen-Prüss, A.B., M.D.	Assistant Professor of Medicine
*Deryl Hart, A.B., A.M., M.D.	Professor of Surgery
*Duncan Charteris Hetherington, A.B., M.A., Ph.D., M.D.	Associate Professor of Anatomy
William Henry Hollinshead, B.A., M.S., Ph.D.	Instructor in Anatomy
*Christopher Johnston, A.B., M.D.	Instructor in Medicine
*Robert Randolph Jones, Jr., A.B., M.D.	Assistant in Surgery
Hyman Mackler, A.B., M.A., Ph.D.	Instructor in Physiology and Pharmacology
William deBerniere MacNider, M.D.	Visiting Lecturer in Special Pharmacology
Elsie Wilson Martin, A.B., M.S.	Professor of Dietetics
Forrest Draper McCrea, M.S., Ph.D.	Associate Professor of Physiology
Ernest Parrish McCutcheon, D.D.S.	Instructor in Dentistry
*Mary H. Muller, R.N.	Instructor in Anesthesiology

* Indicates persons with previous professional training or experience at The Johns Hopkins University.

1. For a complete listing of all members of the faculty of the Duke University Schools of Medicine, Nursing and Health Services during the period 1930–41 see Wilburt C. Davison, *The First Twenty Years*, 104–15.

*William Alexandre Perlzweig, B.S.,
A.M., Ph.D. — Professor of Biochemistry
Elbert Lapsley Persons, A.B., M.D. — Instructor in Medicine
Francis Ross Porter, A.B. — Intern in Hospital Administration
*Mary Alverta Poston, A.M. — Instructor in Bacteriology
*Watson Smith Rankin, M.D. — Lecturer in Public Health
Robert James Reeves, A.B., M.D. — Instructor in Roentgenology
Robert Alexander Ross, B.S., M.D. — Instructor in Obstetrics and Gynecology

Julian Meade Ruffin, A.B., M.D. — Assistant Professor of Medicine
*Alfred Rives Shands, Jr., B.A., M.D. — Instructor in Orthopaedics
*Mildred M. Sherwood — Head Nurse on Pediatric Ward
*David Tillersin Smith, A.B., M.D. — Associate Professor of Medicine
*Susan Gower Smith, A.B., M.A. — Instructor in Biochemistry
*Mary H. Snively, R.N. — Associate in Anesthesiology
*Francis Huntington Swett, A.B., M.A.
Ph.D. — Professor of Anatomy
*Haywood Maurice Taylor, B.S., M.S.,
Ph.D. — Assistant Professor of Biochemistry
Marcellus Eaton Winston — Superintendent of Duke Hospital

Appendix 4. Comparative summary of revenue: Duke University School of Medicine and Hospital, 1930–1941

	1930–31	1931–32	1932–33	1933–34	1934–35	1935–36	1936–37	1937–38	1938–39	1939–40	1940–41
Patient revenue											
Public dispensary	6,042.05	9,441.98	10,165.83	16,597.72	19,270.78	19,826.90	26,945.61	26,047.23	26,346.79	27,623.88	54,079.45
Hospital accounts	136,934.68	112,977.24	111,095.75	204,655.12	263,219.23	302,570.88	379,064.39	415,203.53	452,929.23	508,750.83	586,465.71
The Duke Endowment											
Regular Endowment	360,000.00	360,000.00	314,551.54	219,560.20	338,654.37	373,811.46	360,914.15	442,205.15	495,278.81	531,256.58	546,854.92
Account: free bed patients	9,192.00	34,298.00	53,335.00	55,475.00	57,197.00	69,375.00	72,042.00	62,970.00	74,132.00	73,743.00	77,669.00
For purchase of equipment	110,000.00										
Special gifts			1,063.45	15,555.26							
General Education Board	a	80,000.00	60,000.00	40,000.00	20,000.00						
Medical School tuition	a	67,585.25	76,514.30	81,523.00	86,968.00	96,315.00	102,930.00	107,195.00	115,125.00	115,050.00	115,245.00
Nurses tuition	a	5,050.00	6,000.00	7,200.00	6,800.00	6,600.00	7,600.00	8,075.00	9,650.00	10,260.00	12,535.00
Other student tuition	a					2,346.71	1,007.90	375.00	600.10	1,892.98	1,170.00
Hospital dormitory rents		3,992.00	7,440.77	9,303.22	5,335.62	9,491.44	3,243.85	4,669.00	3,357.01	516.33	
Student rental plan fees						6,984.31	5,518.34	5,251.04	5,348.80	4,281.59	
Duke Pathological Service				6,458.54	7,135.00	900.00	1,725.00	6,280.00	5,917.96	5,486.63	
Lederle Laboratories				65.00	800.00						
Eli Lilly & Company				500.00	500.00						
Susan G. Smith Research							400.00				
Rockefeller Foundation							2,764.39				
Metabolic studies							800.00				
Cremation fees								615.00	250.00		
Miscellaneous funds[c]					5,018.25	7,052.70	2,821.00	105.70	63.23		b23,895.45
Total revenue	622,168.73	673,344.47	640,166.64	657,481.06	810,908.25	895,774.40	967,796.63	1,078,391.65	1,188,998.93	1,278,861.32	1,417,844.53

a. These items (if received) were included in the General Fund of the University.
b. Grant for establishing department of psychiatry.
c. Some research grants were not included either as Medical School or Hospital revenue. Lists of these were published annually in the Duke University *Bulletin* as a part of the annual report of the Medical School and Hospital in "The Report of the President and other Officers."
Note—This table derived from data taken from Duke University Reports on Audit, 1932–1941.

Appendix 5. Comparative statement of expenditures for the Duke University School of Medicine, 1932–1941[a]

	1932–33	1933–34	1934–35	1935–36	1936–37	1937–38	1938–39	1939–40	1940–41
Administration	13,836.69	16,854.22	15,769.57	14,916.65	16,371.38	18,879.94	16,162.69	19,271.22	17,834.36
Animals[b]		3,464.96	4,512.74	4,931.59	4,808.43	8,485.68	9,585.28	11,104.16	10,245.11
Anatomy	25,278.32	21,360.77	28,411.29	30,427.14	33,905.42	35,380.87	35,567.48	38,700.59	40,847.44
Biochemistry	21,968.89	18,763.79	24,093.37	25,351.49	27,789.34	29,055.72	32,284.22	33,218.43	33,009.28
Biological Division[c]							40,878.52	45,331.27	49,687.06
Medicine	52,696.33	50,396.86	62,285.54	72,077.17	77,927.82	84,940.33	56,937.60	61,098.53	60,541.91
Neurology	1,500.00	0	0	0	0	0	0	0	0
Obstetrics	15,824.41	15,354.92	23,241.07	26,851.85	27,891.43	32,200.11	33,225.00	35,517.86	37,103.84
Pathology	24,857.96	21,048.72	20,151.12	26,694.54	27,154.20	31,268.61	33,293.25	35,874.60	38,405.68
Pediatrics	21,291.07	17,235.39	20,591.98	23,305.23	21,504.28	23,747.63	26,000.79	26,153.47	27,539.02
Physiology	22,094.62	20,107.94	25,744.48	28,064.58	29,401.41	30,101.62	35,058.41	36,187.71	38,351.78
Preventive Medicine	300.00	519.18	75.00	0		0	0	0	0
Psychiatry									23,835.45
Surgery	30,477.63	26,149.26	35,348.55	36,733.06	10,347.47	51,171.04	59,215.67	62,732.88	64,625.05
Miscellaneous		7,058.54	11,238.86	14,630.07		6,280.00	5,917.96	5,936.63	4,453.20
Total expenditures (excluding income of clinical departments derived from Private Diagnostic Clinics)	230,549.87	218,314.55	278,463.57	393,983.37	317,371.70	351,511.55	384,166.87	411,127.55	446,479.18

a. The breakdown of expenditures was unavailable for the years 1930–31, and 1931–32, as was the total expenditure for the former; for the latter it was $204,768.26.
b. Prior to 1933–34 the cost of animals for research was included in the expenditures of individual departments.
c. Absorbed into the Department of Medicine.
Note—Data for this table taken from Duke University Reports on Audit, 1932–1941.

Appendix 6. Comparative statement of expenditures, Duke Hospital, 1930–1941

	1930–31	1931–32	1932–33	1933–34	1934–35	1935–36	1936–37	1937–38	1938–39	1939–40	1940–41
Administration											
salaries & wages			19,875.52	22,861.31	29,311.21	30,530.50	31,097.52	31,925.06	34,579.21	30,692.24	34,367.70
other expenses			17,602.79	18,126.76	20,064.81	19,977.19	22,678.79	26,004.81	24,743.73	31,497.82	35,433.95
Totals	$ 34,864.42	40,734.54	37,478.31	40,988.07	49,376.02	50,507.69	53,776.31	57,929.87	59,322.94	62,190.06	69,800.65
Professional care of pts.											
Nursing: salaries & wages	136,723.51	139,716.71	101,083.13	81,556.63	110,991.66	127,903.18	137,672.96	155,510.48	181,586.38	192,503.60	206,866.72
other	a	a	a	5,742.88	6,967.52	9,055.74	10,994.29	12,443.64	29,860.74	33,483.09	32,943.58
Medical service: salaries	69,970.67	46,351.03	37,266.99	13,012.89	15,649.63	14,375.83	15,852.26	17,939.80	22,236.89	22,669.80	26,219.64
pharm. & drugs	a	a	a	a	a	a	a	a	a	a	53,416.46
other supp. & ex.	a	a	a	15,967.16	21,710.01	22,746.74	29,692.02	35,294.73	42,000.42	47,344.26	48,507.47
X-Ray Dept.	15,412.10	17,047.43	20,021.01	18,337.73	22,793.39	25,918.65	30,891.37	32,944.15	35,839.43	41,701.85	58,168.74
Miscellaneous	35,857.77	a	a	20,560.03	27,314.70	29,069.18	32,485.96	38,814.12	46,432.99	45,550.46	a
	a	2,591.28	2,235.30	3,578.42	5,614.91	8,965.37	10,175.54	14,795.18	13,787.31	15,996.67	19,391.23
Totals	$257,964.05	205,706.45	160,706.43	158,755.74	211,041.82	238,063.69	267,764.40	307,742.10	371,744.15	402,249.73	445,513.84
Household expenses											
Housekeeping: salaries	24,997.23	20,609.14	18,194.34	22,981.51	26,679.45	16,673.90	19,566.31	21,692.26	20,113.58	23,794.25	34,699.35
linen, bedding & supp.	a	a	a	a	a	14,236.29	16,147.10	20,145.23	20,307.68	29,123.59	24,336.87
Laundry: salaries	15,338.46	23,925.66	20,145.57	22,299.69	27,637.37	2,329.26	2,522.12	4,078.55	6,346.41	5,682.78	9,928.25
laundry & supplies	a	a	a	a	a	31,864.90	28,707.53	32,196.51	39,679.44	44,703.75	50,606.65
Totals	$ 40,335.69	44,534.80	38,339.91	45,281.20	54,316.82	65,004.35	66,943.06	78,112.55	86,347.11	103,302.37	119,271.12
Plant operation & maintenance											
heat, light, power	39,900.35	46,808.68	50,417.50	45,257.81	55,398.52	57,545.32	58,263.12	62,700.38	63,213.03	60,683.36	67,056.78
replacements and repairs	15,331.41	9,524.14	6,765.84	11,873.14	10,114.06	14,727.07	17,420.35	22,688.39	23,503.87	27,332.68	26,320.43
Totals	$ 55,231.76	56,332.82	57,183.34	57,130.95	65,512.58	72,272.39	75,683.37	85,388.77	86,716.90	88,016.04	93,377.21
Dietary Department											
salaries & wages	27,143.25	26,736.64	27,919.33	27,441.01	34,177.20	36,877.78	38,777.69	44,543.88	46,549.38	49,125.13	56,408.40
food	50,664.53	67,499.94	66,395.99	67,245.60	84,947.84	97,611.61	106,559.51	108,114.11	113,890.89	119,720.96	136,223.12
other	1,878.62	4,205.59	3,500.06	5,366.27	5,833.78	6,091.62	6,273.15	7,238.29	7,491.24	7,789.67	15,594.30
Totals	79,686.40	98,442.17	97,815.38	100,052.88	124,960.82	140,611.01	151,610.35	159,896.28	167,931.51	176,635.76	208,225.82
Public dispensary	12,423.94	11,572.65	10,998.06	12,014.53	18,606.12	21,442.53	27,893.66	29,325.97	27,598.66	30,454.37	30,576.13
Grand totals	$480,506.26	457,323.43	402,521.43	414,223.37	523,814.18	587,907.66	643,671.15	718,395.54	799,661.27	862,846.33	966,764.77

a. Included in above.

Appendix 7. Growth of the faculty of the School of Medicine, 1931–1941

	1931–32	1932–33	1933–34	1934–35	1935–36	1936–37	1937–38	1938–39	1939–40	1940–41
Anatomy	1P, 1AsP	1P, 1AsP	1P, 1AsP	1P, 1AsP	1P, 1AsP 3A	1P, 1AsP 2A	1P, 1AsP 2A	1P, 1AsP 2A	1P, 1AsP 2A&P	1P, 1AsP 2A&P
Biochemistry	1P, 1A&P	1P, 1A&P	1P, 2A&P	1P, 1AsP 1A	1P, 2AsP 1A	1P, 2AsP 1A	1P, 2AsP 2A	1P, 1AsP 2A&P, 2A	1P, 1AsP 3A&P, 1A	1P, 1AsP 2A&P, 1A
Physiology, Pharmacology & Nutrition	1P, 1AsP 1A&P	1P, 1AsP 1A&P	1P, 1AsP 1A&P	1P, 2AsP	1P, 2AsP 1A&P, 1A	1P, 2AsP 1A&P	1P, 2AsP 1A&P	1P, 3AsP	1P, 3AsP 1A	1P, 3AsP 1A
Pathology	1P	1P, 1AsP	1P, 1AsP	1P, 1AsP 1A&P	1P, 1AsP 1A&P	1P, 1AsP 1A&P	1P, 1AsP 1A&P	1P, 1AsP 1A	1P, 1AsP 1A&P	1P, 1AsP 1A&P
Bacteriology		1P	1P	1P, 1A&P 1A	1P, 1A	1P, 1A&P 1A	1P, 1A&P 1A	1P, 1A&P 1A	1P, 1AsP 1A&P	1P, 1AsP 1A&P
Medicine	1P, 2AsP 3A&P	2P, 1AsP 3A&P	1P, 2AsP 4A&P	1P, 1AsP 4A&P, 4A	1P, 1AsP 4A&P, 4A	1P, 1AsP 4A&P, 7A	1P, 3AsP 2A&P, 9A	1P, 3AsP 2A&P, 9A	1P, 3AsP 2A&P, 9A	1P, 2AsP 2A&P, 8A
Surgery	1P, 3A&P	1P, 3AsP 2A&P	1P, 3AsP 3A&P	1P, 3AsP 3A&P	1P, 5AsP 1A&P	1P, 5AsP 2A&P, 2A	1P, 5AsP 3A&P,13A	1P, 5AsP 3A&P, 3A	1P, 5AsP 4A&P, 6A	1P, 4AsP 5A&P, 5A
Roentgenology	1A&P	1AsP	1AsP	1AsP	1AsP	1AsP	1AsP	1AsP	1AsP	1AsP, 1A
Obstetrics and Gynecology	1P, 2A&P	1P, 1AsP 1A&P	1P, 1AsP 1A&P	1P, 1AsP 1A&P	1P, 1AsP 1A&P	1P, 1AsP 1A&P	1P, 2AsP 1A&P	1P, 2AsP 1A&P	1P, 2AsP 2A&P	1P, 2AsP 2A&P
Pediatrics	1P	1P, 1A&P	1P, 1A&P	1P, 1A&P	1P, 1A&P 1A	2P, 1A&P 1A	1P, 1A&P 1A	1P, 2A&P 1A	1P, 2A&P 1A	1P, 2A&P 1A
Preventive Medicine and Public Health										1P, 1A
Zoology		1P	1P	1P	1P	1P	1P	1P	1P	1P
Neuropsychiatry	(Department separated from department of medicine.)									1P, 1AsP 1A&P, 2A
Total	23	28	32	38	44	50	55	58	64	66

a. Members of the faculties of the associated schools, instructors, fellows, assistants, and lecturers not included. Code: P = professor, AsP = associate professor, A&P = assistant professor, A = associate (rank first created 1934).
Note—Data from Duke University *Bulletin*, 1932–41.

Notes

Chapter 1: The Agricultural-Industrial Frontier: Durham, 1865–1889

1. Hiram V. Paul, *History of the Town of Durham, N.C.* Population statistics from William K. Boyd, *The Story of Durham*, p. 97; Nannie May Tilley, *The Bright-Tobacco Industry*, p. 551.
2. The accounts of Sherman and Johnston, agreeing in all but the smallest details, are found in William T. Sherman, *Memoirs of General William T. Sherman*, 2:348–67; and Joseph E. Johnston, *Narration of Military Operations*, pp. 399–420. See also George W. Pepper, *Personal Recollections of Sherman's Campaigns in Georgia and the Carolinas*, pp. 405–22.
3. Paul, 25–26; John G. Barrett, *Sherman's March Through the Carolinas*, pp. 253–54, 263–66. See also J. D. Cameron, *A Sketch of the Tobacco Interests in North Carolina*, p. 43.
4. James A. Robinson, "William Thomas Blackwell" (Undated and unpublished biographical sketch in the Charles Leonard Van Noppen Papers). Cameron, p. 52; *Raleigh News and Observer*, 5 April 1896, p. 12; Boyd, pp. 57–76; Paul, pp. 102–4; Tilley, pp. 549–55.
5. Paul, pp. 50–77; Boyd, pp. 62–67.
6. *Raleigh News and Observer*, 5 April 1896, p. 12.
7. Samuel A. Ashe, ed., *Biographical History of North Carolina*, 3: 85–87, Boyd, p. 81; Paul, pp. 15–52. John W. Jenkins, *James B. Duke: Master Builder*, pp. 44–48. *Raleigh News and Observer*, 5 April 1896, pp. 9, 16. *Raleigh Morning Post*, 27 Dec. 1903, p. 2. Joseph C. Robert, *The Tobacco Kingdom*, pp. 222–23.
8. Paul, pp. 50–77.
9. *Raleigh News and Observer*, 5 April 1896, p. 16; Tilley, p. 533; Joseph C. Robert, *The Story of Tobacco in America*, p. 140.
10. Jenkins, 58–60; George W. Watts to Eugene Morehead, 31 July 1899, Eugene Morehead Papers; Tilley, p. 525.
11. Boyd, p. 76.
12. Robert, *Story of Tobacco*, p. 140; Tilley, p. 509; Jenkins, p. 65. The North Carolina tobacco industry of these years is described in detail in Paul, pp. 158–209.
13. Robert, *Story of Tobacco*, p. 141; Tilley, pp. 557–58; Jenkins, p. 68.
14. Edward F. Small, "The Correct Version of the Beginnings of a Trust" undated typescript, pp. 4–7, W. Duke Sons & Co. to E. F. Small, 10 March 1884, James B. Duke to E. F. Small, 20 March 1884, Edward Featherston Small Papers. *The Durham Sun*, 26 April 1921, p. 5.
15. W. Duke Sons & Co. to E. F. Small, 11 April 1884, Edward F. Small Papers.
16. Paul, pp. 207–09. U.S. Bureau of Corporations, *Report of the Commissioner of Corporations on the Tobacco Industry*, 1:63.
17. Tilley, pp. 572–75; Small, p. 16; U.S. Bureau of Corporations, *Report*, 1:64.
18. W. Duke Sons & Co. to E. F. Small, 23 May 1884 and 20 Oct. 1884, Edward F. Small Papers.

19. W. Duke Sons & Co. to E. F. Small, 4 Oct. 1884, Edward F. Small Papers. Jenkins, p. 73. John K. Winkler, *Tobacco Tycoon*, pp. 57–58. *Raleigh News and Observer*, 5 April 1896, p. 16.
20. Paul, p. 78. North Carolina State Board of Health, *Biennial Report . . . to the General Assembly of North Carolina; Session 1877*, table insert between pp. 26 and 27. *Bulletin of the North Carolina Board of Health*, 1, no. 3 (June 1886): 23; no. 4 (July 1886): 32. Summaries of monthly reports from Durham's health officers and mortuary statistics are found in the *Bulletin*. "Minutes of the Board of Commissioners of the Town of Durham," E (18 Sept. 1883): 13. Title varies, especially after Durham was incorporated as a city; cited hereafter as MBCD. Boyd, pp. 209–10.
21. MBCD, E (18 Sept. 1883): 11. *Bulletin of the N.C. Board of Health*, 2, no. 5 (Aug. 1887): 44.
22. MBCD, E (16 Dec. 1884–3 April 1888): 49–294; *The Durham Tobacco Plant*, 5 Aug. 1885, p. 2; *The Daily Tobacco Plant*, 13 July 1888, p. 1; 13 Oct. 1888, p. 1.
23. North Carolina State Board of Health, *Second Biennial Report . . . to the General Assembly of North Carolina, Session 1889*, pp. 66–72.
24. *The Durham Tobacco Plant*, 8 Feb. 1888, p. 3.
25. *The Daily Tobacco Plant*, 7 July 1888, p. 1.
26. *The Durham Tobacco Plant*, 15 Feb. 1888, p. 3; 29 Feb. 1888, p. 3. *Bulletin of the North Carolina Board of Health*, 3, no. 1 (April 1888): 136; no. 2 (May 1888): 149; no. 4 (July 1888): 199; no. 7 (Oct. 1888): 209. *Raleigh Morning Post*, 27 Dec. 1903, p. 2.
27. *The Daily Tobacco Plant*, 7 July 1888, p. 1; 13 July 1888, p. 3.
28. *The Durham Tobacco Plant*, 20 July 1888, p. 5.
29. *The Daily Tobacco Plant*, 15 Nov. 1888, p. 1; 16 Nov. 1888, p. 1; 17 Nov. 1888, p. 1; 19 Nov. 1888, p. 1; 23 Nov. 1888, p. 1; 3 Dec. 1888, p. 1. Boyd, p. 117.
30. George W. Watts to E. F. Small, 16 Dec. 1885; James B. Duke to E. F. Small, 27 Jan. 1886, Edward F. Small Papers. See especially the letterheads, which advertised the capitalization.
31. Tilley, pp. 519, 575–76; Boyd, p. 89–90.
32. Tilley, pp. 575–76; George W. Watts to E. F. Small, 12 July 1887; 25 July 1887, Edward F. Small Papers; W. M. Morgan to Eugene Morehead, 9 March 1888; 15 Dec. 1888; 7 Feb. 1889, Eugene Morehead Papers.
33. Tilley, p. 577; Jenkins, p. 84.

Chapter 2: The American Medical Revolution: Medicine at Trinity? 1889–1923

1. *The Daily Tobacco Plant*, 25 May 1889, p. 1.
2. Nora Chaffin, *Trinity College, 1839–1892: The Beginnings of Duke University. Annual Register of Trinity College*, 1890–91:15.
3. John Franklin Crowell, *A Program of Progress: An Open Letter to the General Assembly of North Carolina of 1891*.

4. John Franklin Crowell, *Personal Recollections of Trinity College, North Carolina: 1887–1894*, pp. 99–100.
5. John Franklin Crowell, "The Removal of Trinity College," *Raleigh Christian Advocate*, 26 June 1889, p. 1; 3 July 1889, p. 1. Crowell's undated "Plan of a Methodist University in North Carolina" is among the Trinity College Papers, Nov.–Dec. 1890. See also *Trinity Archive*, 1 (June 1888) : 152.
6. J. W. Alspaugh to J. F. Crowell, 21 Aug. 1889, Trinity College Papers. See also Earl W. Porter, *Trinity and Duke, 1892–1924*, pp. 20–22; Chaffin, p. 491.
7. Chaffin, pp. 494–504.
8. Crowell, *Personal Recollections*, pp. 162–67.
9. *Transactions of the Medical Society of the State of North Carolina*, 9 (1858) : 18–22; 26 (1880) : 6–7. Cited hereafter as *Transactions*. J. Howell Way and L. B. McBrayer, *Medical Colleges in North Carolina*, pp. 136–37; William W. McLendon, "Edenborough Medical College."
10. "Minutes of the Board of Trustees of the University of North Carolina, with Minutes of the Executive Committee," 29 Jan. 1879. Cited hereafter as "U.N.C. Minutes." Kemp B. Battle, *History of the University of North Carolina*, 2:166–67.
11. *Transactions*, 37 (1890) : 5.
12. "U.N.C. Minutes," 30 Nov. 1888; 27 Feb. 1889; 20 Feb. 1890; 11 Feb. 1891. See also R. H. Whitehead to Kemp Battle, 2 Sept. 1899 and 7 Sept. 1899, University Papers, Wilson Library, U.N.C.
13. *Transactions*, 37 (1890) : 5.
14. *State Chronicle* in *Raleigh Christian Advocate*, 25 March 1891, p. 3.
15. U.S. Bureau of the Census, *Fourteenth Census of the United States: 1920. Population*, 3:20. R. G. Leland, *Distribution of Physicians in the United States*, p. 6. *Transactions*, 38 (1891) : 75–76.
16. *State Chronicle*, 24 March 1891; *Raleigh Christian Advocate*, 25 March 1891; *State Chronicle*, 1 April, 1891. Way and McBrayer, pp. 150–51.
17. Crowell's manuscript (dated 7 April 1891) containing this plan is found among the Trinity College Papers.
18. Crowell, *Personal Recollections*, p. 180; *Transactions*, 38 (1891): 10–13, 83–84; Way and McBrayer, p. 153; Chaffin, pp. 503–16; Porter, pp. 29–32.
19. A detailed report of the expansion of the American Tobacco Company is found in U.S. Bureau of Corporations, *Report*, 1:1–196. Statistics on the increased volume of cigarette sales which provided Duke and his associates with the funds to build the American Tobacco Company are found in William W. Young, *The Story of the Cigarette*, p. 115. The American Tobacco Company, *"Sold American!"—The First Fifty Years*, pp. 20–40.
20. Unsigned article, "Benjamin Newton Duke," Ashe, *Biographical History of North Carolina*, 3:97; S. A. Ashe, "George Washington Watts," Ashe, 1: 474–79; S. A. Ashe, "Julian Shakespeare Carr," Ashe, 2:51–60. Boyd, pp. 120–22, 138–46.
21. *Raleigh News and Observer*, 5 April 1896, p. 16; U.S. Bureau of the Census, *Fourteenth Census of the United States: 1920. Population*, 1:120. S. A. Ashe, "Lewis Albert Carr," Ashe, 5:55–58; Tilley, pp. 636–37; Boyd, p. 128.

22. Tilley, pp. 405–16. B. N. Duke Papers, 1893.
23. B. N. Duke to J. B. Cobb, 4 Oct. 1894, B. N. Duke Papers.
24. B. N. Duke to J. F. Crowell, 14 June 1890, Trinity College Papers. B. N. Duke to J. W. Alspaugh, 17 May 1892; B. N. Duke to E. A. Yates, 14 Oct. 1892. The arrangement by which B. N. Duke administered the family's local philanthropy is revealed in B. N. Duke to J. B. Duke, 29 Dec. 1893, B. N. Duke Papers.
25. J. F. Crowell to B. N. Duke, 22 Nov. 1892, Trinity College Papers. "Minutes of the Board of Trustees of Trinity College and Duke University," 7 June 1893. Cited hereafter as "Minutes, Duke Trustees." B. N. Duke to James B. Duke, 10 Nov. 1894, B. N. Duke Papers. Porter, pp. 37, 49; Crowell, *Personal Recollections*, pp. 41–42; Paul N. Garber, *John Carlisle Kilgo*, pp. 94–122.
26. Boyd, p. 211.
27. Charles L. Van Noppen, ed., *In Memoriam: George Washington Watts*, pp. 6–7.
28. "Presentation speech of Mr. Geo. W. Watts, presenting the first Watts Hospital to the citizens of Durham, North Carolina, February 22, 1895." Typescript copy in possession of Albert Carr, Durham, North Carolina. Opened in 1889, the Johns Hopkins Hospital already was recognized as the model hospital in America. *Annual Report of the Trustees, Watts Hospital*, p. 10; Van Noppen, pp. 26–29; Boyd, pp. 211–17; *Durham Recorder*, 16 April 1900, p. 7.
29. "Minutes of the Trustees of Watts Hospital," 1 Jan. 1895, 7 Feb. 1895; *Annual Report of the Trustees, Watts Hospital*, pp. 5–6.
30. MBCD, H: 544–46; Boyd, p. 217; *The Durham Globe*, 11 July 1895, p. 3.
31. Statements of B. N. Duke's account with J. E. Stagg for the months May–November 1901 show ten separate checks under the heading "colored hospital" totalling $5,404.60, B. N. Duke Papers; Boyd, pp. 219–22.
32. *Durham Recorder*, 6 April 1900, pp. 1, 7, 11–12; Van Noppen, pp. 8–9; B. R. Lacy, Jr., *George W. Watts: The Seminary's Great Benefactor;* W. Duke to R. Shepard, 4 June 1900; B. N. Duke to J. E. Underwood, 11 July 1900; B. N. Duke to Bishop Haid, 18 June 1900; B. N. Duke to J. W. Jenkins, 5 Nov. 1900, B. N. Duke Papers.
33. John Carlisle Kilgo, *The Lines of the Future Development of Trinity College*, pp. 3–11.
34. Porter, pp. 147–64.
35. Ibid., pp. 225–26.
36. Joseph E. Griffin, "The Buzzard Roost Case," pp. 5–9.
37. Durham, North Carolina, Chamber of Commerce, *Durham, North Carolina*, p. 4; *Durham Directory, 1907–1908*, pp. 8–9. John Sprunt Hill, "Remarks on the History of Watts Hospital."
38. Telegrams, Joseph Graham to B. N. Duke, 20 Sept. 1909; Duke to Graham, 20 Sept. 1909, Trinity College Papers.
39. John C. French, *A History of the University Founded by Johns Hopkins*, pp. 106–13, 417–25.
40. French, p. 112.
41. "Minutes, Duke Trustees," 22 Nov. 1909.
42. "Minutes, Duke Trustees," 7 June 1897; Garber, p. 110.

43. Quoted in Robert H. Woody, ed., *The Papers and Addresses of William Preston Few,* p. 29.

44. Woody, pp. 46–60; Porter, pp. 96–141; "Report of the Treasurer of Trinity College, June 1, 1910," p. 9, Trustee Records.

45. Few-Buttrick correspondence, 27 Oct. 1910–10 June 1911; E. C. Sage to Few, 31 Jan. 1916; Few–E. C. Sage correspondence, Nov.–Dec. p. 1920; Few to J. G. Brown, 3 July 1922, Few Papers; Porter, pp. 163, 171–72, 180–81, 189–90, 211–12.

46. Abraham Flexner, "Medical Education in the United States and Canada," *Carnegie Foundation for the Advancement of Teaching Bulletin,* no. 4, pp. viii–x, 12, 153 (map), 279–82; Abraham Flexner, *I Remember,* pp. 112–32.

47. Few to Simon Flexner, 18 March 1916, Few Papers.

48. Abraham Flexner to Few, 22 March 1916, 15 Dec. 1917; Few to General Education Board, 12 Dec. 1917, Few Papers.

49. William P. Few, "The Beginnings of an American University" (unpublished, ca. 1940), ch. 1, p. 2, Few Papers. Porter, p. 184.

50. *University of North Carolina Record,* no. 171 (Dec., 1919); p. 57; no. 183 (Dec. 1920), pp. 55–56.

51. Raymond B. Fosdick, *Adventure in Giving: The Story of the General Education Board,* pp. 161–68.

52. Few, "Beginnings of an American University," ch. 7, pp. 1–2; Interview with W. T. Laprade, 20 April 1967.

53. "Reasons for Locating the Government Hospital in Durham," undated, Few Papers; "U.N.C. Minutes," 27 Jan. 1920.

54. Letters among the papers of John Sprunt Hill, Watts's executor, show the same fourfold pattern of giving to schools, churches, hospitals, and orphanages earlier adopted both by him and the Duke family. John Sprunt Hill Papers, 25 March 1921.

55. Few to E. C. Sage, 15 Feb. 1921, Few Papers; "Appendix to the Report of the President to the Board of Trustees of Trinity College," 21 June 1921, Trustee Records; Few to John Sprunt Hill, 22 July 1921; Few to Mrs. G. W. Watts, 22 July 1921; Few to W. S. Rankin, 13 Aug. 1921; Few to Abraham Flexner, 10 Oct. 1921, 10 Nov. 1921, Few Papers.

56. Quoted in Woody, p. 98.

57. "U.N.C. Minutes," 9 Dec. 1921.

58. "U.N.C. Minutes," 23 March 1922, 1 June 1922; *Transactions,* 69 (1922): 321–27; Louis R. Wilson, *The University of North Carolina, 1900–1930,* pp. 559–61.

59. Few to Abraham Flexner, 19 May 1922; Flexner to Few, 22 May 1922, Few Papers.

60. Chase to Zebulon Judd, 26 June 1922; Chase to H. M. London, 12 July 1922, University Papers.

61. "Four Year Medical School and State Hospital," 22 Oct. 1922, University Papers.

62. The Chamber of Commerce, Charlotte, North Carolina, *Charlotte as the Location of the Clinical Years of the Medical School of North Carolina.* Harry W. Chase to W. N. Everett, 2 Nov. 1922, University Papers.

63. W. N. Everett to Chase, 20 Sept., 1922; Chase to Everett, 22 Sept. 1922, University Papers; J. H. Way to Few, 23 Oct. 1922, Few Papers.
64. Few to B. N. Duke, Dec. 1922, quoted in Woody, p. 99.
65. "U.N.C. Minutes," 20 Dec. 1922; "The North Carolina Medical College," undated, Few Papers.
66. Few to B. N. Duke, 20 Dec. 1922, quoted in Woody, pp. 100–01; Few to Abraham Flexner, 20 Dec. 1922, Few Papers.
67. William P. Few, "As to a Medical School in North Carolina," undated memo; Few to C. W. Toms, 17 Jan. 1923, Few Papers; *Raleigh News and Observer*, 20 Dec. 1922–18 Jan. 1923; *Durham Morning Herald*, 21 Dec. 1922–18 Jan. 1923.
68. E. C. Brooks to Few, 11 Jan. 1923; H. W. Chase to Few, 18 Jan. 1923, Few Papers; H. W. Chase to Governor Cameron Morrison, 18 Jan. 1933, University Papers.
69. Few to B. N. Duke, 27 Jan. 1923, Few Papers.
70. "Report of the Committee on the Four Year Medical School," 25 Jan. 1923, University Papers; "U.N.C. Minutes," 9 Feb. 1923; Few to John Sprunt Hill, 8 Feb. 1923, Few Papers; H. W. Chase to Albert Coster, 13 March 1923, University Papers; Wilson, p. 568.
71. Few to B. N. Duke, 27 Jan. 1923; Few to Abraham Flexner, 22 Jan. 1923, Few Papers.
72. Few to C. W. Toms, 30 Jan. 1923, 23 March 1923, Few Papers.
73. Few to J. W. Long, 23 March 1923, Few Papers.
74. *Transactions*, 70 (1923) : 234–39.
75. Charles M. Strong, *History of Mecklenburg County Medicine*, pp. 79–80.
76. *Transactions*, 71 (1924) : 92–95. See also Harry W. Chase, "Medical Education," p. 116.
77. Few, "The Beginnings of An American University," ch. 7, p. 6, Few Papers.

Chapter 3: Natural Resources Supporting Social Services: The Duke Endowment, 1923–1927

1. Few, "The Beginnings of an American University," ch. 1, pp. 2–3, Few Papers.
2. James B. Duke to J. J. Eads, 10 Jan. 1925, Few Papers.
3. Winkler, p. 290; Wilburt C. Davison, *The Duke University Medical Center, 1892–1960*, pp. 2–3.
4. Porter, p. 227.
5. Jenkins, p. 27.
6. *Durham Morning Herald*, 27 Jan. 1924, p. 2; Claude W. Munger, *Report of a Study of the Lincoln Hospital*, p. 23.
7. Winkler, p. 290.
8. William R. Perkins, *An Address on The Duke Endowment: Its Origin, Nature, and Purposes*, p. 4.
9. *Durham Morning Herald*, 13 Dec. 1924, p. 1.
10. The plan, perhaps the original draft, is among Few's papers. He called it "Initial Steps toward Foundation of D.U."

11. Davison, *The Duke University Medical Center,* p. 2.
12. R. G. Leland, *Distribution of Physicians in the United States,* pp. 2, 6.
13. Lewis Mayers and Leonard V. Harrison, *The Distribution of Physicians in The United States,* pp. 71–72, 189, 191, 193–94.
14. A. H. Sands, Jr., to Few, 27 Oct. 1923, Few Papers.
15. Davison, *The Duke University Medical Center,* p. 2. For Rankin's views on the cooperative medical school see Raleigh *News and Observer,* 28 Dec. 1922, p. 1.
16. Interview with Watson S. Rankin by Frank Rounds, 11 Jan. 1965.
17. W. S. Rankin, "Plan for a System of Hospitals," undated, Few Papers.
18. Watson S. Rankin to Dr. M. M. Seymour, 10 Aug. 1925, Rankin Papers.
19. Watson S. Rankin, "Statement by W. S. Rankin, M.D., at the request of Mr. Alex H. Sands, Jr., of the Duke Foundation, prepared in February, 1924," Few Papers.
20. Porter, pp. 230–31.
21. The summary in the following paragraphs is from Paul Clark, *James Buchanan Duke and the Saugenay Region of Canada,* pp. 145–74, 191–94.
22. Interview with Norman A. Cocke, by Frank Rounds, 20 April 1963, typescript in Duke Endowment Collection, Perkins Library, Duke University.
23. *Indenture of James B. Duke Establishing The Duke Endowment, With Provisions of the Will and a Trust of Mr. Duke Supplanting the Same.* Cited hereafter as *The Duke Endowment.*
24. Few to J. L. Jackson, 16 Nov. 1925, Few Papers.
25. Porter, pp. 232–37.
26. "Last Will and Testament of James B. Duke," p. 8, James B. Duke Papers. Cited hereafter as "Will."
27. "Will," p. 23. By a codicil dated 1 Oct. 1925 he later changed this item to provide $7,000,000 for building at Duke University, ten percent of the income from the remainder for support of Duke University, and ninety percent for expenditure under the hospital provision. *The Duke Endowment,* p. 51; Porter, p. 234.
28. Few to Mary L. Wyche, 21 May 1925, Few Papers.
29. *Durham Morning Herald,* 3 Sept. 1925, p. 12.
30. Few to James Dowd, 9 March 1925; Few to F. S. Aldridge, 30 June 1925, Few Papers. Details of the construction of these buildings is found in Alex H. Sands, Jr., "The Duke Endowment: Report of the Secretary, 1925 and 1926," pp. 3–4, Flowers Papers.
31. Winkler, p. 301.
32. Jenkins, pp. 258–60. Controversy over the exact cause of Mr. Duke's death continued for some years, at least one authority holding that he died of an aregeneratory anemia. George F. Minot to F. M. Hanes, 21 March 1945, Duke Endowment Collection.
33. *Durham Morning Herald,* 5 Oct. 1925.
34. U.S., *Statutes at Large,* 43, Pt. 1:303–06; W. P. Few to Wallace Buttrick, 7 Dec. 1925; W. R. Perkins to Furnifold M. Simmons, 8 Dec. 1925, Few Papers; *Durham Morning Herald,* 8 Dec. 1925, p. 6.
35. U.S., Congress, House, *Reports,* 69th Cong., 1st sess., 1926, H. Rept. 356, pp. 7–11; U.S., *Statutes at Large,* 44, pt. 2:70–73; Few Papers, 13 Nov. 1925–19 Feb. 1926.

36. Alex H. Sands, Jr., "The Duke Endowment: Report of the Secretary" (1925), pp. 3–4, Flowers Papers.
37. George G. Allen to Horace Trumbauer, 9 April 1926, Few Papers.
38. Few to Abraham Flexner, 28 June 1926, Few Papers.
39. Few to Buttrick, 3 Feb. 1926; Buttrick to Few, 6 Feb. 1926, Few Papers; Few quoted in Davison, *The Duke University Medical Center*, p. 5.
40. Few, "The Beginnings of an American University," ch. 7, p. 8.
41. Few to Abraham Flexner, 28 June 1926, 22 Jan. 1927, Few Papers.
42. *Annual Report of the General Education Board, 1926–1927*, p. 5; Few to C. W. Toms, 17 Sept. 1926; Few to Trevor Arnett, 24 Nov. 1926; Few to W. R. Perkins, 13 Jan. 1930, Few Papers.
43. Lewis H. Weed to Few, 13 March 1926; Few to Weed, 15 March 1926; Few to James R. Angell, 30 June 1926, Few Papers.
44. Cornell's reports are among the Few Papers. See also William B. Bell to Few, 27 Jan. 1926, Few Papers.
45. *Durham Morning Herald*, 14 Oct. 1926, p. 13; 13 Nov. 1926, p. 7.
46. Rankin to Few, 20 Nov. 1926; Few to Rankin, 22 Nov. 1926, Few Papers.
47. Few to W. H. Welch, 17 Jan. 1927, Few Papers.
48. Quoted in Davison, *The Duke University Medical Center*, p. 7. Davison's telegram is among the Few Papers.

Chapter 4: Imprint of an Education: The Building, 1927–1931

1. *Journal of the Florida Medical Association* (March 1954): 647; Biographical Memo, "Davison, Wilburt Cornell," Few Papers; interview with Wilburt C. Davison, by Frank Rounds, May 1964.
2. Wilburt C. Davison, "Sir William Osler, Reminiscences," pp. 110, 113; interview with W. C. Davison, May, 1964.
3. Wilburt C. Davison, "The 1915 Serbian Typhus Epidemic."
4. Davison, "Sir William Osler, Reminiscences," p. 113; Wilburt C. Davison, "The Diagnosis of Enteric Fever (Typhoid and Paratyphoid A and B) by Agglutination Test"; interview with W. C. Davison, May 1964.
5. Davison, "Sir William Osler, Reminiscences," pp. 114–22; W. C. Davison, "John Howland."
6. Davison, "Sir William Osler, Reminiscences," pp. 122–25. Davison to John Howland, 12 Nov. 1918; Davison to John Howland, 27 Feb. 1919, Davison Collection, Duke Medical Center Library.
7. Davison, "John Howland," pp. 484–86; John Howland to W. C. Davison, 10 Aug. 1920; Harvey Cushing to W. C. Davison, 22 Feb. 1927, Davison Collection; personal interview with Dr. David T. Smith, 10 Jan. 1969.
8. G. G. Allen to Few, 20 Jan. 1927; W. S. Rankin to Few, 22 Jan. 1927; W. deB. MacNider to Few, 22 Jan. 1927; W. T. Parrott to Few, 4 Feb. 1927, Few Papers; *Durham Morning Herald*, 14 Feb. 1927, p. 5.
9. G. G. Allen to Few, 20 Jan. 1927; Few to Davison, 4 Feb. 1927, Few Papers.
10. William Blackburn, *The Architecture of Duke University*, pp. 1–16; W. C. Davison, "The Duke University School of Medicine," p. 35; Davison, *The Duke University Medical Center*, pp. 11–12, 17.

11. W. W. Brierly to Few, 2 March 1927; Few to G. G. Allen, 4 March 1927; Allen to Few, 14 March 1927; Few to W. R. Perkins, 13 Jan. 1930, Few Papers.
12. W. C. Davison to Few, 22 March 1927; 30 March 1927; 17 May 1927; W. C. Davison to Abraham Flexner, 19 Sept. 1927, Few Papers.
13. *Durham Morning Herald,* 15 March 1927, p. 1.
14. Davison to Few, 22 March 1927, Few Papers.
15. Davison, "The Duke University School of Medicine," pp. 35–36; *Raleigh News and Observer,* 20 April 1927, p. 2.
16. Wilburt C. Davison, "The Selection of Medical Students," pp. 955–58; W. C. Davison, "The Significance of Present Entrance Requirements"; W. C. Davison, "An M.D. Degree Five Years After High School," pp. 1812–14; W. C. Davison, "Two Additional Years in College Versus Two More Years in Hospital"; Davison, "The Duke University School of Medicine," p. 36.
17. W. C. Davison, "Liberalizing the Curriculum"; C. C. Bass, "Demands on the Medical Practitioner in the South During One Year."
18. Davison, "The Duke University School of Medicine," p. 36; Davison, "An M.D. Degree Five Years After High School," p. 1815.
19. Davison, "The Duke University School of Medicine," pp. 36–39.
20. Few to Davison, 27 April 1927; Davison to Few, 17 May 1927, Few Papers.
21. Davison to Few, 27 May 1927, Few Papers.
22. Few to G. G. Allen, 20 June 1927, Few Papers.
23. Few to W. S. Rankin, 16 Sept. 1927, Few Papers.
24. Few to C. W. Toms, 15 Sept. 1927; W. C. Davison to A. Flexner, 19 Sept. 1927; W. C. Davison to Few, 20 Sept. 1927, Few Papers.
25. *Durham Morning Herald,* 3 Oct. 1927, p. 5; Davison, *The Duke University Medical Center,* pp. 15–17.
26. *Durham Morning Herald,* 4 Nov. 1927, p. 9; 20 Nov. 1927, p. 6; 16 Dec. 1927, p. 2.
27. *Durham Morning Herald,* 16 Dec. 1927, p. 2; 4 June 1928, p. 5; 25 Oct. 1928, p. 1; W. C. Davison, "The Duke University School of Nursing," 24 Oct. 1928, Davison Papers.
28. "Minutes of the Meetings of The Duke Endowment Building Committee," Oct. 28, 1927, Flowers Papers. Hereafter cited as "Building Committee Minutes." N. A. Cocke to R. L. Flowers, 8 Nov. 1927, Department of Plant Engineering and Maintenance Repairs Papers.
29. A. C. Lee to James Q. Davis, 11 Dec. 1929, Flowers Papers.
30. A. C. Lee to Flowers, 12 March 1929, Few Papers.
31. "Minutes to the Meetings of the Stockholders of Duke Construction Company," 12 Nov. 1927, Department of Plant, Engineering and Maintenance Papers. Hereafter cited as "Construction Company Minutes." "Building Committee Minutes," 28 Oct. 1927.
32. Alex H. Sands, Jr., "The Duke Endowment: Report of the Secretary, 1928" pp. 3–4, Flowers Papers; Duke Construction Company, "Statement of Estimated Costs, Expenditures, and Obligations as of Dec. 31, 1931," Department of Plant, Engineering and Maintenance Papers.
33. "Minutes, Duke Trustees," 21 March 1928.
34. Interview with A. C. Lee, by Frank Rounds, April 1963.
35. A. P. Leighton, Jr., to Davison, 1 Aug. 1928; Charles B. Keisler to Davi-

son, 29 Aug. 1928; U. W. Preston to Davison, 21 June 1930; I. D. Metzger to Davison, 24 Sept. 1928, Davison Papers.

36. R. L. Flowers to Alex H. Sands, Jr., 3 Aug. 1928, 10 Sept. 1928; R. L. Flowers to W. C. Davison, 16 April 1928, Flowers Papers.

37. W. C. Davison to R. L. Flowers, 11 Nov. 1928, Few Papers; *Durham Morning Herald*, 25 July 1928, p. 2.

38. Louis S. Reed, *The Ability to Pay for Medical Care*, p. 16.

39. Davison to Few, 27 May 1927, Few Papers; *The Duke Endowment: Year Book*, no. 1 (1924–1928), p. 21.

40. Pierce Williams, *The Purchase of Medical Care Through Fixed Periodic Payment*, pp. 239–44.

41. W. C. Davison, "Hospital Insurance, a plan for the organization of Hospital Associations in North and South Carolina," 20 Sept. 1928, Davison Papers.

42. Davison, "Hospital Insurance."

43. Davison to Watson S. Rankin, 11 Aug. 1928, Davison Papers.

44. W. C. Davison to George B. Crenshaw, 3 Oct. 1928; Davison to Dr. Moore, 24 Oct. 1928; Davison to H. L. Amoss, 18 Dec. 1928, Davison Papers.

45. *Durham Morning Herald*, 14 March 1929, p. 9.

46. Davison to H. F. Kleinfelter and Co., 5 Sept. 1928; Louis I. Dublin to Davison, 20 Nov. 1929; Davison to Stuart Graves, 24 Feb. 1931; J. G. Brothers, "An Outline History of the Hospital Care Association of Durham, North Carolina," unpublished term paper dated 17 May 1946, Davison Papers.

47. *Durham Morning Herald*, 19 Aug. 1928, sec. 4, p. 1.

48. Davison, *The Duke University Medical Center*, p. 16. "Building Committee Minutes," 28 Aug. 1928.

49. W. C. Davison, "Address before the N.C. Hospital Association," 18 May 1928, Davison Papers; "Building Committee Minutes," 25 Sept. 1928.

50. W. C. Davison to Few, 2 Jan. 1928, Few Papers.

51. The master lists of candidates for positions are dated, and show Davison working on this two-year plan, with the clinical department considered first. See lists for surgery, dated 1 Feb. 1929; internal medicine, 13 Feb. 1929, pathology, 13 Feb. 1929 as compared to anatomy, 29 Dec. 1929 and pharmacology, 29 Dec. 1929, Davison Papers; Davison to Few, 2 Jan. 1929; Richard M. Pearce to Davison, 18 March 1929, Few Papers; Memo, "Duke University School of Medicine: Information for Pre-Medical Students" (1929?), Davison Papers.

52. Richard H. Shryock, *The Unique Influence of the Johns Hopkins University on American Medicine*, p. 63; Davison, *The Duke University Medical Center*, p. 21.

53. Undated biographical sketch, "Harold L. Amoss," Davison Papers.

54. Davison to H. L. Amoss, 27 Nov. 1928, 3 Dec. 1928, Davison Papers.

55. H. L. Amoss to Davison, 17 Dec. 1928, Davison Papers.

56. Davison, *The Duke University Medical Center*, p. 23.

57. See Davison Papers, 2–6 Feb., 1929.

58. W. C. Davison to H. L. Amoss, 30 Jan. 1929, Davison Papers.

59. *Durham Morning Herald*, 16 March 1929, pp. 1–2.

60. Davison to Ashley Weech, 6 Nov. 1928, Davison Papers. The vote is

recorded in *Journal of the Association of American Medical Colleges*, 4 (Jan. 1929) : 32.

61. Bessie Baker to W. C. Davison, 25 Nov. 1928; K. H. Van Norman to Davison, 20 Feb. 1928, Davison Papers. Davison, *The Duke University Medical Center*, p. 23.

62. W. C. Davison to H. L. Amoss, 26 Feb. 1929; Amoss to Davison, 4 March 1929; Davison to J. D. Hart, 15 March 1929; Davison to Bessie Baker, 29 April 1929, Davison Papers.

63. W. C. Davison to H. L. Amoss, 18 Dec. 1928, Davison Papers.

64. W. C. Davison to H. L. Amoss, 15 May 1929, 23 April 1929; Davison to Bessie Baker, 4 May 1929, Davison Papers.

65. See Davison's correspondence with H. L. Amoss and J. D. Hart and Bessie Baker, March–Sept. 1929, Davison Papers; "Building Committee Minutes," 25 Sept. 1928, 29 April 1929, Flowers Papers.

66. Davison to H. L. Amoss, 7 Jan. 1929, Davison Papers.

67. W. C. Davison to H. L. Amoss, 30 April 1929; Amoss to Davison, 4 May 1929, Davison Papers.

67. W. C. Davison to H. L. Amoss, 30 April 1929; Amos to Davison, 4 May 1929, Davison Papers.

68. W. C. Davison to J. D. Hart, 4 Sept. 1929, Davison Papers; Davison, *The Duke University Medical Center*, pp. 20–26.

69. Davison Papers, April 1929. See especially correspondence to and from J. D. Hart and H. L. Amoss. Davison, *The Duke University Medical Center*, pp. 24–25.

70. H. L. Amoss to W. C. Davison, 24 May 1929; 6 Nov. 1929; Davison to Amoss, 1 Nov. 1929; J. D. Hart to Davison, 4 Sept. 1929, Davison Papers. *Durham Morning Herald*, 20 July 1930, p. 13.

71. W. C. Davison to H. L. Amoss, 27 May 1929, Davison Papers.

72. W. C. Davison, *The First Twenty Years*, p. 41; J. D. Hart to W. C. Davison, 1 June 1929; see also the list of book dealers approached, Davison Papers.

73. W. C. Davison to R. M. Pearce, 8 March 1929, Few Papers; R. M. Pearce to Davison, 18 March 1929; Trevor Arnett to W. P. Few, 10 April 1929, Few Papers.

74. Few to Trevor Arnett, 22 April 1929, Few Papers; William Preston Few, *The Duke Endowment and Duke University*, pp. 5–8.

75. W. C. Davison to Trevor Arnett, 22 April 1929, Few Papers.

76. Telegram, Trevor Arnett to W. P. Few, 9 Nov. 1929, Few Papers.

77. Few to C. W. Toms, 27 Nov. 1929, Few Papers; *Annual Report of the General Education Board, 1929–1930*, p. 41.

78. "Minutes, Duke Trustees," 2 June 1930.

79. Davison to Few, 9 March 1929–3 Jan. 1931, Few Papers.

80. W. C. Davison to H. L. Amoss, 23 Dec. 1929; 7 Feb. 1930; 24 March 1930, Davison Papers, *Durham Morning Herald*, 20 July 1930, p. 13. Interview with W. C. Davison, by Frank Rounds, April 1964.

81. J. D. Hart to W. C. Davison, 17 Feb. 1930; 28 March 1930, 3 May 1930; W. C. Davison to H. L. Amoss, 23 Dec. 1929; 22 Jan. 1930, Davison Papers; Davison, *The First Twenty Years*, pp. 104–05; *Durham Morning Herald*, 20 July 1930, p. 13.

82. W. C. Davison to H. L. Amoss, 22 Jan. 1930; 10 Feb. 1930; 17 Feb. 1930; Amoss to Davison, 4 March 1930, Davison Papers; *Durham Morning Herald*, 20 July 1930, p. 13.

83. Davison to H. L. Amoss, 14 May 1929; 16 Dec. 1929; 24 Dec. 1929, Davison Papers.

84. W. P. Few to W. R. Perkins, 3 Jan. 1930, Few Papers.

85. Davison, *The Duke University Medical Center*, p. 21.

86. Ibid., pp. 33–34.

87. W. C. Davison to H. L. Amoss, 23 Jan. 1930; Amoss to Davison, 25 Jan. 1930, Davison Papers.

88. W. C. Davison to Bessie Baker, 24 May 1929; 29 Aug. 1929; Baker to Davison, 10 June 1929, Davison Papers. *Bulletin of Duke University*, 2, no. 1 (Jan. 1930) : 18–19.

89. "Wilburt Cornell Davison," undated biographical sketch in the files of the Director of the Duke University Hospital.

90. *Durham Morning Herald*, 12 May 1929, sec. 4, p. 1; Blackburn, *The Architecture of Duke University*, pp. 65–66.

91. *Durham Morning Herald*, 19 Jan. 1930, p. 5.

92. *Durham Morning Herald*, 19 Jan. 1930, p. 5; 13 April 1930, p. 5; W. C. Davison to H. L. Amoss, 26 Sept. 1929, Davison Papers.

93. W. C. Davison to John Q. Meyers, 9 May 1930, Davison Papers. Attached is a leaflet entitled "Duke Hospital and Out-Patient Clinic, Durham, North Carolina," designed for distribution to all physicians in the Carolinas and Virginia, which gave details of the hospital's schedules of hours and charges. See also *Durham Morning Herald*, 13 July 1930, sec. 2, p. 1.

94. *Durham Morning Herald*, 14 June 1930, p. 12; 21 July 1930, pp. 1–2; W. P. Few to Charles C. Jarrell, 22 July 1930, Few Papers.

95. Davison, *The Duke University Medical Center*, p. 19.

96. W. P. Few to W. R. Perkins, 7 Aug. 1930, Few Papers.

97. *Durham Morning Herald*, 22 July 1930, p. 12.

98. Duke University Hospital Accessions Book, 1:1–18.

99. Duke University Hospital Operation Book, 1:1–4.

100. Davison, *The Duke University Medical Center*, pp. 27–28.

101. Duke University Hospital Accessions Book, 1:1–18.

102. The Duke Endowment, Hospital Section, "Application for Assistance, Duke University, 1931," Duke Endowment Papers. These percentages are taken from figures covering the period 21 July 1930–31 Dec. 1930.

103. W. P. Few to W. R. Perkins, 7 Aug. 1930, Few Papers.

104. "Minutes of the Executive Committee of the Faculty of the Duke University School of Medicine," 1 Sept. 1930; hereinafter cited as "Executive Committee Minutes"; W. C. Davison to John T. Bauer, 15 Jan. 1931, Davison Papers; "Minutes, Duke Trustees," 2 June 1930; Davison, *The First Twenty Years*, p. 3.

105. Interview with Wiley D. Forbus, 2 June 1965; interview with David T. Smith, 17 Sept. 1965; interview with Robert J. Reeves, 7 March 1967, videotapes in possession of Department of Audiovisual Education, Duke University Medical Center.

106. Davison, *The Duke University Medical Center*, p. 35.

107. "Executive Committee Minutes," 3 Feb. 1931; Paul F. Clark, *The University of Wisconsin Medical School: A Chronicle, 1848–1948*, pp. 32–35.
108. "Executive Committee Minutes," 3 March 1931, 7 April 1931; interview with Dr. J. Lamar Callaway, 4 June 1969.
109. Duke Hospital Accessions Book, 1, July 1930–April 1931.
110. Duke University Payroll Sheets, 1930–1931.
111. Interview with Wiley D. Forbus, Durham, N.C., 2 June 1965; "Executive Committee Minutes," 1 Sept. 1930, 5 Nov. 1930, 1 Dec. 1930.
112. "Executive Committee Minutes," 7 April 1931; W. C. Davison, "Duke University School of Medicine and the Duke Hospital," working copy dated 9 April 1931, Davison Papers; Duke Hospital Accessions Book, 1, January-April 1931; W. P. Few to G. G. Allen, 4 April 1931, Few Papers.
113. *Durham Morning Herald*, 1 May 1930, p. 1, 19 April 1931, p. 7.
114. "Dedication of the Duke University School of Medicine and Hospital," pp. 1099–113, 1121–24; *Durham Morning Herald*, 24 April 1931, pp. 1–2.
115. "Dedication of the Duke University School of Medicine and Hospital," pp. 1116–21.

Chapter 5: Experiments in Cooperation: Financing Medicine During the Depression Decade

1. Cleon C. Mason, "Are Hospital Costs Too High?," p. 59; I. S. Falk, "An Introduction to National Problems in Medical Care."
2. Ray L. Wilbur, "The Relationship of Medical Education to the Cost of Medical Care."
3. For a bibliography on this issue as reflected in the popular press see *The First Two Years' Work of the Committee on the Cost of Medical Care* pp. 21–23. See especially Watson S. Rankin," "Economics of Medical Service," and Michael M. Davis, "Problems of Health Service for Negroes."
4. Frank G. Dickinson and James Raymond, *The Economic Position of Medical Care, 1929–1953*, pp. 8, 31.
5. *Medical Care for the American People*, pp. 9–10.
6. I. S. Falk, C. Rufus Rorem, and M. D. Ring, *The Costs of Medical Care*, pp. 136–49, 200–10; *Medical Care for the American People*, p. 18.
7. Interdepartment Committee to Coordinate Health and Welfare Activities, *The Nation's Health*, p. 11; W. F. Walker, "What The Depression Has Done to Health Service."
8. Reed, pp. 79–96.
9. *The Five-Year Program of The Committee on the Cost of Medical Care*, p. 6.
10. *Medical Care for the American People*, pp. 58–71, 104–44. Falk, et al., pp. 346–66, 397–434, 437–513, 573–77.
11. Memo, "Annual University Subsidies to the School of Medicine and Duke Hospital," Davison Papers; The Duke Endowment, Hospital Section, "Application For Assistance, Duke University Hospital," 1931, p. 1.
12. The Duke Endowment, Hospital Section, "Application For Assistance, Duke University," 1930, pp. 2–3; 1931, 2–3.

13. Interview with Dr. Julian M. Ruffin, 15 Jan. 1969; The Duke Endowment Hospital Section, Applications for Assistance, Duke University, 1930–1940; F. M. Hanes, "Memo to Dr. Hart," 21 June 1935, F. M. Hanes Papers; Duke University, Durham, North Carolina, Reports on Audit, 1932–1940.

14. Interview with F. Vernon Altvater, 21 Dec. 1968.

15. Interview with Dr. Julian M. Ruffin, 15 Jan. 1969; Davison to M. M. Davis, 28 May 1931, Davison Papers.

16. Willis B. Blue and Wilburt C. Davison, "The Evolution of Infant Feeding and the Advantages and Disadvantages of Soured Milk Mixtures."

17. "Minutes of the Meetings of the Trustees of the Duke Endowment," 6 (28 Nov. 1933) : 32–34; Altvater and Davison to Rankin, 11 Dec. 1936, Duke Endowment Papers; Davison, *The First Twenty Years,* pp. 58–59.

18. Interview with Dr. J. Deryl Hart, 16 Dec. 1968; interview with Dr. David T. Smith, 10 Jan. 1969; J. Deryl Hart, "The Responsibility of the Medical Profession to Medical Education," p. 601.

19. Interview with Dr. David T. Smith, 10 Jan. 1969; Hart, "The Responsibility of the Medical Profession to Medical Education," p. 601.

20. Interview with Dr. David T. Smith, 10 Jan. 1969.

21. Hart, "The Responsibility of the Medical Profession to Medical Education," p. 601; W. C. Davison, "The Duke Private Diagnostic Clinic," p. 482.

22. Interview with Dr. David T. Smith, 10 Jan. 1969.

23. Interview with Dr. David T. Smith, 10 Jan. 1969; interview with Dr. Julian M. Ruffin, 15 Jan. 1969.

24. Undated memo, no title; undated memo, "The Origin and Development of the Anna H. Hanes Research Fund," F. M. Hanes Papers; interview with Dr. Julian M. Ruffin, 15 Jan. 1969.

25. Undated memo, "The Origin and Development of the Anna H. Hanes Research Fund," F. M. Hanes Papers.

26. Interview with Dr. J. Deryl Hart, 16 Dec. 1968; Hart, "The Responsibility of the Medical Profession to Medical Education," p. 617.

27. Interview with Dr. David T. Smith, 10 Jan. 1969.

28. Davison, "The Duke Private Diagnostic Clinic," p. 483. For a somewhat different salary policy developed at a state university by a Hopkins-trained dean see Clark, pp. 36–39.

29. Interview with Dr. J. Deryl Hart, 16 Dec. 1968; Hart, "The Responsibility of the Medical Profession to Medical Education," pp. 601–02.

30. Interview with Dr. J. Deryl Hart, 16 Dec. 1968; interview with Dr. David T. Smith, 10 Jan. 1969.

31. Interview with Dr. J. Deryl Hart, 16 Dec. 1968.

32. Davison, *The First Twenty Years,* p. 7.

33. Interview with Dr. J. Deryl Hart, 16 Dec. 1968.

34. Hart, "The Responsibility of the Medical Profession to Medical Education," p. 602; interview with Dr. David T. Smith, 10 Jan. 1969.

35. Davison to Lewis H. Weed, 23 Jan. 1932, Davison Papers.

36. F. Vernon Altvater to W. C. Davison, 1 Oct. 1932, Davison Papers; F. Vernon Altvater, "Flat Rates for 4½ Years," p. 47; "Minutes, Duke Trustees," 8 June 1931.

37. F. Vernon Altvater, "Theory and Application of Inclusive or Flat Rate

Plans," p. 63; see also R. G. Hils, "Prices, Business Activity and War," p. 96.

38. Letters introducing Altvater to officials of medical schools and clinics in Illinois, Iowa, Colorado, and Minnesota are filed under the dates of 6 June–19 July 1932, among the Davison Papers. Davison, *The First Twenty Years*, p. 46.

39. Altvater to Davison, 13 July 1932, 1 Oct. 1932, Davison Papers. The proposal Altvater presented to Davison on October 1 was later published, in a generalized form, in F. Vernon Altvater, "A Flat Rate Plan Designed to Help Both Hospital and Patient."

40. Altvater to Davison, 1 Oct. 1932, Davison Papers; Altvater, "A Flat Rate Plan Designed to Help Both Hospital and Patient," pp. 72–75.

41. Rankin to Altvater, 29 Oct. 1932, Davison Papers.

42. William A. Perlzweig, Memo, "The Altvater Plan"; Altvater to Davison, 1 Oct. 1932, Davison Papers.

43. Perlzweig to Davison, 7 March 1933, Davison Papers; Hugh T. Lefler, *History of North Carolina*, 2:772, 791. Lefler's figures for the year 1933 as a whole, however, show that in North Carolina both cash farm income and income payments to individuals rose, which tended to increase the number of persons able to make some payment toward the cost of their care.

44. Davison-Rankin correspondence, 1 March 1933–6 April 1933; memo, "Duke Hospital, 1932," Davison Papers.

45. Interview with Dr. David T. Smith, 10 Jan. 1969.

46. Memo, "Duke Hospital Rates Effective for April 18, 1933," Flowers Papers; Davison to Flowers, undated; Altvater to Davison, 1 Oct. 1932, Davison Papers.

47. Davison to Rankin, 31 Aug. 1933, Davison Papers.

48. *Greensboro Daily News*, 20 Nov. 1933, p. 2.

49. D. B. McCrary (President, Randolph Hospital, Inc., Asheboro, N.C.) to Rankin, 20 Nov. 1933; Rankin to Davison, 21 Nov. 1933, Davison Papers.

50. Rankin to McCrary, 21 Nov. 1933; Rankin to Davison, 5 Dec. 1933; Memo, "The Policy of Duke Hospital," 2 April 1934, Davison Papers.

51. Davison to Rankin, 6 Dec. 1933, Davison Papers.

52. *Southern Medicine and Surgery*, 95 (Dec. 1933) : 675.

53. Davison to Rankin, 14 March 1934, Davison Papers.

54. Dr. O. L. Miller (Charlotte), to Davison, 5 April 1934; Dr. J. Street Brewer (Roseboro, N.C.), to F. Ross Porter, 23 April 1934; Graham L. Davis to Davison, 17 March 1934, Davison Papers.

55. F. Ross Porter, "What is a Charity Patient," working copy dated 17 April 1934, Davison Papers.

56. "Minutes, Duke Trustees," 4 June 1934.

57. Memo, "Duke Hospital—1933," Davison Papers.

58. W. C. Davison to D. W. Sorrell, 15 March 1933; Memo, "The Duke Hospital, 1932"; Davison to W. S. Rankin, 14 June 1934, Davison Papers.

59. *Durham Morning Herald*, 30 July 1932, p. 3; 30 Dec. 1932, p. 3; 10 June 1933, p. 12; 1 July 1933, p. 12, 9 Aug. 1933, p. 1.

60. MBCD, R (19 June 1933) : 230; *Durham Morning Herald*, 20 June 1933, p. 8; 1 July 1933, p. 12.

61. *Durham Morning Herald,* 14 June 1933, sec. 2, p. 8; 16 June 1933, p. 5.
62. MBCD, R (19 March 1934): 318, 321; R (2 April 1934): 328; R (21 May 1934): 334; *Durham Morning Herald,* 20 March 1934, p. 3; Davison to W. S. Rankin, 14 June 1934, Davison Papers.
63. *Durham Morning Herald,* 8 June 1934, sec. 1, p. 4; sec. 2, p. 4; 11 June 1934, p. 4.
64. *Durham Morning Herald,* 2 June 1934, p. 14; 7 June 1934, p. 8; 8 June 1934, sec. 2, p. 4.
65. *Durham Morning Herald,* 12 June 1934, sec. 2, p. 8.
66. *Durham Morning Herald,* 12 June 1934, sec. 2, p. 8; 3 July 1934, sec. 2, p. 8; 18 Aug. 1934, p. 12; 23 Oct. 1934, p. 12; "Minutes of the Meetings of the Board of Commissioners of Durham County, N.C.," (25 July 1934): 474.
67. MBCD, R (7 Jan. 1935): 391–92; R (4 Feb. 1935): 399; *Durham Morning Herald,* 8 Jan. 1935, p. 3.
68. Memo, "Duke Hospital, July 21, 1930–December 31, 1933"; Memo, "Duke Hospital, 1938," Davison Papers.
69. Altvater, "Flat Rates for 4½ Years," pp. 47–48.
70. Memo, "Duke Hospital, 1938," Davison Papers.
71. F. Vernon Altvater to D. W. Newsom, 30 Sept. 1937, Davison Papers; Altvater, "Flat Rates for 4½ Years," p. 48.
72. "Suggested Operating Methods for the Duke University Medical Guild," 26 Oct. 1932; "Duke University Medical Guild," 15 Nov. 1932, Davison Papers.
73. "Suggested Duke University Medical Guild," 3 Nov. 1932; "Discussion of Insurance Plan, Faculty Club Meeting, November 1st, 1932," Davison Papers.
74. Graham L. Davis, "Hospital Insurance—Why Not?"; Graham L. Davis, "Principles that Should Govern the Development of Group Hospitalization in North Carolina," 24 April 1934, Duke Endowment Papers.
75. "Minutes of the Meetings of the Board of Directors of the Hospital Care Association, Incorporated," 28 April 1934; hereinafter cited as "Care Directors' Meetings"; Altvater to Rankin, 26 Jan. 1937, North Carolina Blue Cross-Blue Shield Papers; J. G. Brothers, "An Outline History of the Hospital Care Association of Durham, North Carolina," unpublished term paper dated 17 May 1946, p. 20, Davison Papers; Lewis S. Reed, *Blue Cross and Medical Service Plans,* pp. 10–11; Wilburt C. Davison, "The Birth of Blue Cross."
76. Donald E. Deichmann to Trustees of The Duke Endowment, 24 Jan. 1936; Certificate issued to Charles L. Medlin and wife, 22 Sept. 1933, by The Hospital Care Association, Inc., North Carolina Blue Cross-Blue Shield Papers; Brothers, pp. 20–21; *Sunday Herald Sun,* Durham, N.C., 5 Nov. 1933, p. 12; E. M. Herndon to Walter J. McNerney, 28 Jan. 1965, North Carolina Blue Cross-Blue Shield Papers. For a general description of this and similar plans see C. Rufus Rorem, *Hospital Care Insurance,* pp. 6–46.
77. "Care Directors' Meetings," 28 April 1934. A notebook among The North Carolina Blue Cross-Blue Shield Papers, showing claims and disbursements from 16 Jan. 1934, to 3 Oct. 1934, clearly shows that subscribers among the Duke staff and faculty filed far more claims than other Association members.

78. Elisha M. Herndon, "Early History of the Hospital Care Association, Incorporated," unpublished paper, 1968, in possession of author, p. 25.
79. "Care Directors' Meetings," 11 Feb. 1935; 16 Feb. 1935; 22 Dec. 1936.
80. Altvater to Alex H. Sands, Jr., 17 Dec. 1936; Deichmann to Davison, undated, North Carolina Blue Cross-Blue Shield Papers; Brothers, pp. 21–26.
81. Altvater to Rankin, 26 Jan. 1937, North Carolina Blue Cross-Blue Shield Papers.
82. J. T. Richardson, "The Origin and Development of Group Hospitalization in the United States, 1890–1940," pp. 24–25; *Durham Morning Herald,* 18 July 1935, p. 9. For the public discussion of this movement see *Durham Morning Herald,* 18 July 1935, p. 9. For the public discussion of this movement see *Durham Morning Herald,* 18 July 1935, p. 9; *The Charlotte Observer,* 11, 13 July, 4, 5, 18 Oct. 1934; *Charlotte News,* 24 June, 15, 25 July 1934; *Greensboro Daily News,* 15 July 1934; *Asheville Citizen-Times,* 29 July, 1 Aug. 1934; *Winston Daily Free Press,* 27 July 1934.
83. The Duke Endowment, Hospital Section, "Application for Assistance from the Joint Committee on Group Hospitalization of the North Carolina Hospital Association and the Medical Society of the State of North Carolina," 3 Jan. 1935, Flowers Papers.
84. F. Ross Porter, undated memo, "Hospital Prepayment in North Carolina," Davison Papers; W. C. Davison, "The Birth of Blue Cross"; W. S. Rankin to R. L. Flowers, 8 March 1935, Flowers Papers; Eugene B. Crawford, *A History of Hospital Saving Association of North Carolina, Inc.* For an enthusiastic running commentary on the development of Hospital Saving Association see *Southern Hospital,* vol. 3 (April, 1935), vol. 6 (May, 1938).
85. "Care Executive Committee Minutes," 23 May 1937; interview with George Watts Hill, 20 Nov. 1968; "Hospitalization Insurance"; Felix A. Grisette, *The Second Year: Annual Report of the Executive Director of Hospital Saving Association for the Year 1937,* p. 2.
86. Rorem, "Approved List of Hospital Care Insurance Plans," p. 80; Rorem to Rankin, 12 May 1937, Duke Endowment Papers; telegram, Rorem to B. R. Roberts, 24 May 1938, copy in North Carolina Blue Cross-Blue Shield Papers; George Watts Hill, Memo, "Hospital Care Association," 17 Dec. 1938, North Carolina Blue Cross-Blue Shield Papers; Brothers, pp. 33–34. For the role of the American Hospital Association in the establishment of hospital service plans see Reed, pp. 14–15; Richardson, pp. 22–23, 29–33; for interest of other states see Rankin to M. W. Whitaker (Lynchburg, Va.), 8 April 1938; Rankin to Dr. John A. Chase, Jr. (University of South Carolina), 29 April 1938, Duke Endowment Papers.

Chapter 6: Learning by Doing: The Training of Duke Physicians

1. Duke Indenture, pp. 23–24.
2. Davison, "Liberalizing the Curriculum," pp. 983–87.
3. Wilburt C. Davison, "Qualities Which a Medical Student and Physician Should Have or Develop."

4. Wilburt C. Davison, "The Future of Medical Education"; interviews with Dr. Wiley D. Forbus, 16 May 1969 and Dr. G. S. Eadie, 20 June 1969.
5. Based on a study of the records of those admitted to the freshman classes of 1930, 1931, 1938 and 1939, in the Recorder's Office, Duke University School of Medicine.
6. "Medical Education in the United States and Canada," pp. 568–69.
7. Wilburt C. Davison, "Changes in Medical Education and Patient Care," p. 181.
8. Council on Medical Education and Hospitals of the American Medical Association, "Medical Education in the United States and Canada," p. 699; Fred C. Zapffe, "Analysis of Entrance Credentials of the Freshman Class, 1931–1932," pp. 42–43.
9. John E. Deitrich and Robert C. Berson, *Medical Schools In the United States at Mid-Century*, p. 238.
10. H. G. Weiskotten and Harold Rypins, "Duke University School of Medicine" (20–23 April 1935), an official accreditation survey report made for the American Medical Association. Copy in files of the Assistant Dean for Student Affairs, Duke University Medical Center.
11. Interview with Dr. Duncan C. Hetherington, 21 May 1969.
12. Francis H. Swett, "Report of the Department of Anatomy—July 1, 1931 to July 1, 1932," Francis H. Swett Papers, Duke University Medical Center Library.
13. Interview with Dr. Duncan C. Hetherington, 26 May 1969.
14. Ibid.
15. Interview with Dr. Warner L. Wells, 19 June 1969.
16. Weiskotten and Rypins, pp. 9–12.
17. Interview with Dr. Mary L. C. Bernheim, 21 May 1969.
18. Interview with Dr. Frederick Bernheim, 21 May 1969.
19. Interview with Dr. George S. Eadie, 20 June 1969.
20. Weiskotten and Rypins, p. 14.
21. Interviews with Dr. David T. Smith, 15 May 1969, and Dr. Elbert L. Persons, 22 May 1969.
22. Weiskotten and Rypins, pp. 17–18.
23. David T. Smith, "Teaching Bacteriology as a Function of the Department of Medicine."
24. Interview with Dr. Elbert L. Persons, 22 May 1969.
25. Wiley D. Forbus, "Report of the Department of Pathology," 22 Sept. 1933, Wiley D. Forbus Papers.
26. Interview with Dr. Wiley D. Forbus, 16 May 1969.
27. Wiley D. Forbus, "Southern Pathological Conference Protocol," 1933, Wiley D. Forbus Papers.
28. Roger D. Baker, "Case Method and Clerkship in Teaching Pathology," pp. 165–71.
29. Roger D. Baker, "Criticism of the General Course in Pathology at Duke School of Medicine, 1933–34," 25 March 1934, Forbus Papers. Included with this report is a file of the students' reactions to the course.
30. Francis H. Swett, "Report of the Department of Anatomy, July 1, 1933 to June 30, 1934," Francis H. Swett Papers; Roger D. Baker, "Criticism of the General Course in Pathology . . . ," Forbus Papers; Weiskotten and Rypins, pp. 14–15.

31. Weiskotten and Rypins, pp. 22–24.
32. Julian M. Ruffin, "A New Method of Teaching Physical Diagnosis."
33. Weiskotten and Rypins, pp. 32–39.
34. *Bulletin of Duke University*, 8 (June 1936) : 264.
35. Harvey Cushing, *The Life of Sir William Osler*, 1:440, 552.
36. Interview with Dr. David T. Smith, 15 May 1969; interview with Dr. Julian M. Ruffin, 20 May 1969.
37. Interview with Dr. J. Lamar Callaway, 3 June 1969.
38. Weiskotten and Rypins, pp. 28, 33, 38, 40.
39. Interview with Dr. Elbert L. Persons, 22 May 1969.
40. The pencil sketches are in the Oscar C. E. Hansen-Pruss Papers.
41. Interview with Dr. Elbert L. Persons, 22 May 1969.
42. Interview with Dr. David T. Smith, 15 May 1969.
43. Interviews with Dr. David T. Smith, 15 May 1969 and Dr. Elbert L. Persons, 22 May 1969.
44. Interview with Dr. J. Deryl Hart, 14 May 1969.
45. Interview with Dr. Robert A. Ross, 12 March 1969.
46. Interview with Dr. J. Lamar Callaway, 29 June 1969.
47. Interview with Dr. F. Bayard Carter, 15 May 1969.
48. Weiskotten and Rypins, p. 41.
49. Wilburt C. Davison, "The Future of American Pediatrics," p. 810.
50. Wilburt C. Davison, *The Compleat Pediatrician*, p. iii.
51. Interview with Dr. Angus McBryde, 23 June 1969.
52. Wilburt C. Davison, "Pediatric Diagnosis."
53. Frederic M. Hanes and Wilburt C. Davison, "Postgraduate Medical Education and Internships," p. 372.
54. The formal protest is among the Davison papers. See also "Executive Committee Minutes," 24 May 1932.
55. Hanes and Davison, p. 373.
56. Interviews with Dr. J. Deryl Hart, 14 May 1969; Dr. David T. Smith, 15 May 1969; Dr. Elbert L. Persons, 22 May 1969.
57. Interview with Dr. Wiley T. Forbus, 16 May 1969.
58. Interview with Dr. J. Deryl Hart, 14 May 1969.
59. Many of the conferences were published in the *North Carolina Medical Journal,* as a post-graduate teaching aid for the physicians of the state. See, for example, "Duke Hospital Clinico-Pathological Conference, November 8, 1939."
60. Interview with Dr. J. Lamar Callaway, 3 June 1969; Dr. Warner L. Wells, 19 June 1969.
61. Davison, *The First Twenty Years*, p. 3.
62. Wilburt C. Davison, "The Future of Medical Education," p. 226.
63. Interview with Dr. Frederick Bernheim, 21 May 1969.
64. Francis H. Swett, "Report of the Department of Anatomy, July 1, 1931 to July 1, 1932," Swett Papers; interview with Dr. George S. Eadie, 20 June 1969.
65. Interview with Dr. Wiley T. Forbus, 16 May 1969; Francis H. Swett, "Report of the Department of Anatomy, July 1, 1932 to June 30, 1933," Swett Papers.
66. Robert K. Merton, "Some Preliminaries to a Sociology of Medical Educa-

tion," in Robert K. Merton, George G. Reader, and Patricia L. Kendall, eds., *The Student Physician,* pp. 22–23.

67. Smith, "Teaching Bacteriology as a Function of the Department of Medicine," pp. 734–35.
68. Interview with Dr. Julian Deryl Hart, 14 May 1969.
69. *Durham Morning Herald,* 28 May 1931, p. 1; 24 July 1931, p. 5; 2 April 1933, p. 3; 12 Aug. 1933, p. 12; 3 March 1934, p. 12.
70. Wiley T. Forbus and John S. Bradway, "Medicolegal Investigation."
71. A sample moot court problem is contained in John S. Bradway, "Duke Legal Aid Clinic Annual Report," 1 June 1939, pp. 5–6, Duke University Archives.
72. Haywood M. Taylor and John S. Bradway, "The Teaching of Legal Medicine."
73. Interview with Dr. Angus McBryde, 23 June 1969.
74. Wilburt C. Davison, "The First Ten Years of the Duke University School of Medicine and Hospital," pp. 528–29.
75. Wilburt C. Davison, "Rural General Practice in Groups," p. 182.
76. The Commission on Graduate Medical Education, *Graduate Medical Education,* pp. 101–02.
77. The Commission on Medical Education, *Final Report of the Commission on Medical Education,* pp. 17–20, tables.
78. Davison, "First Ten Years . . . ," p. 531.
79. *Bulletin of Duke University,* 8, no. 1 (Oct. 1940) : 106–07.
80. Davison, *The First Twenty Years,* p. 73.
81. Davison, "First Ten Years . . . ," p. 527.
82. A. M. Lassek, "The Role of the Southeastern Schools of Medicine in the National Distribution of Physicians."
83. Of 49 practicing graduates born in the Carolinas, 34 remained in the two states to practice, although less than half were general practitioners. *Bulletin of Duke University,* 8, no. 1 (Oct. 1940) : 106–07; Wilburt C. Davison, "Opportunities in the Practice of Medicine."
84. "Minutes, Duke Trustees," 1 June 1935.

Chapter 7: Bringing the Laboratory to the Clinic: Patterns of Research, 1930–1940

1. Francis H. Swett, "Supplement to the Report of the Department of Anatomy, 1933–34," Swett Papers; interview with Dr. George S. Eadie, 20 June 1969.
2. Davison to W. B. Bell, 21 July 1932; Archie S. Woods to Davison, 5 June 1939; R. A. Lambert to F. M. Hanes, 2 June 1941, Davison Papers.
3. A complete bibliography of research published from the Duke University School of Medicine may be compiled from the "Reports of the President and Other Officers," *Bulletin of Duke University* (1931–1941), passim.

4. David T. Smith, "Pellagra—An Historical Review," in Julian M. Ruffin, et al., *Selected Papers*, 1:131. See aso T. Z. Cason, "The Progress of Medical Research in the South."

5. Milton Terris, ed., *Goldberger on Pellagra*, pp. 3–16. This volume contains Goldberger's most important papers and a complete bibliography of his work on the disease.

6. David T. Smith and Julian M. Ruffin, "The Use of Liver Extracts in the Treatment of Pellagra," p. 509. This article contains a full description of the disease; Smith, "Pellagra—An Historical Review," p. 131.

7. David T. Smith, "Discussion," *Southern Medicine and Surgery*, 94 (March 1932) : 134.

8. Smith and Ruffin, "The Use of Liver Extracts in the Treatment of Pellagra," p. 510.

9. Susan Gower Smith, "A New Symptom Complex in Vitamin G Deficiency in Rats."

10. David T. Smith, E. L. Persons, and H. I. Harvey, "On the Identity of Goldberger and Underhill Types of Canine Blacktongue."

11. H. I. Harvey, D. T. Smith, E. L. Persons, and M. V. Burns, "The Effect of Various Fractions of Liver on Experimental Canine Blacktongue."

12. Carl Voegtlin, "Recent Work on Pellagra." This article contains a useful history of the investigations on pellagra from 1735–1920; Ruffin and Smith, "Pellagra Therapy," pp. 105–06.

13. Ruffin and Smith, "The Treatment of Pellagra with Certain Preparations of Liver," pp. 512–21.

14. Julian M. Ruffin and David T. Smith, "A Clinical Evaluation of the Potency of Various Extracts of Liver in the Treatment of Pellagra"; J. M. Ruffin, E. L. Persons, H. I. Harvey, and D. T. Smith, "Evidence for the Existence of Two Factors Necessary for the Successful Treatment of Pellagra or Experimental Canine Black Tongue."

15. David T. Smith and Julian M. Ruffin, "Pellagra Therapy," p. 103; Julian M. Ruffin and David T. Smith, "Studies on Pellagra at the Duke University School of Medicine," Seale Harris, *Clinical Pellagra*, pp. 194–95.

16. Ibid.

17. Ruffin and Smith, "Pellagra Therapy," p. 103.

18. Ruffin and Smith, "The Treatment of Pellagra with Certain Preparations of Liver," p. 514; Ruffin and Smith, "Pellagra Therapy," p. 104.

19. David T. Smith and Julian M. Ruffin, "Effect of Sunlight on the Clinical Manifestations of Pellagra."

20. Interview with Dr. D. T. Smith, 14 Feb. 1969; for samples of the progress charts compiled on each patient see Ruffin and Smith, "The Treatment of Pellagra with Certain Preparations of Liver," pp. 517–18.

21. W. J. Dann, "Nicotinic Acid and Vitamin B_2."

22. C. A. Elvehjem, R. J. Madden, F. M. Strong, and D. W. Woolley, "Relation of Nicotinic Acid and Nicotinic Amide to Canine Black Tongue"; C. A. Elvehjem, R. J. Madden, F. M. Strong and D. W. Woolley, "The Isolation and Identification of the Anti-Blacktongue Factor." The latter article contains a useful history of nicotinic acid.

23. David T. Smith and Julian M. Ruffin, "Pellagra Successfully Treated with Nicotinic Acid."

24. Ruffin and Smith, "Studies on Pellagra at the Duke University School of Medicine," pp. 222–23.
25. G. Margolis, L. H. Margolis and S. G. Smith, "The Cure of Experimental Blacktongue and Optimal and Minimal Doses of Nicotinic Acid."
26. Julian M. Ruffin and David T. Smith, "Treatment of Pellagra with Special Reference to the Use of Nicotinic Acid"; Ruffin and Smith, "Studies on Pellagra at the Duke University School of Medicine," p. 241.
27. David T. Smith, Julian M. Ruffin, G. Margolis, and L. H. Margolis, "Treatment of Experimental Canine Blacktongue and Clinical Pellagra with Coramine," p. 775.
28. L. H. Margolis, G. Margolis and S. G. Smith, "Secondary Deficiency of Vitamin B₂ and Riboflavin in the Blacktongue Producing Diet."
29. W. A. Perlzweig, E. D. Levy and H. Sarett, "On Quantitative Determination of Nicotinic Acid and its Derivatives in Urine."
30. Sir Henry Dale, "Chemical Ideas in Medicine and Biology," in *Lilly Research Laboratories: Dedication,* pp. 23–24.
31. David T. Smith and Donald S. Martin, "Blastomycosis"; interview with D. T. Smith, 24 Feb. 1969. For a complete description of this disease see Donald S. Martin and David T. Smith, "Blastomycosis: A Review of the Literature."
32. David T. Smith, "Diagnosis and Treatment of Common Fungus Infections of the Lungs"; David T. Smith, "Diagnosis and Treatment of Fungus Infections in North Carolina."
33. Donald S. Martin, "Complement-Fixation in Blastomycosis"; Donald S. Martin and David T. Smith, "Blastomycosis: A Review of the Literature," p. 288.
34. A case history (Case 4) of this patient is included in Donald S. Martin and David T. Smith, "Blatomycosis: A Report of Thirteen New Cases," pp. 493–95.
35. Smith, "Diagnosis and Treatment of Fungus Infections in North Carolina," p. 601.
36. Interview with Dr. David T. Smith, 24 Feb. 1969; Martin and Smith, "Blastomycosis: A Review of the Literature," p. 289.
37. Martin and Smith, "Blastomycosis: A Review of the Literature," pp. 293–98; Martin and Smith, "Blastomycosis: A Report of Thirteen New Cases," pp. 505–13.
38. Donald S. Martin and N. F. Conant, "A Comparative Study of Nineteen Strains of Blastomyces Dermatitidis Gilchrist and Stokes, 1898."
39. Martin and Smith, "Blastomycosis: A Report of Thirteen New Cases," pp. 511–13; interview with David T. Smith, 24 Feb. 1969.
40. See, for example, Robert L. Peck, Donald S. Martin, and Charles R. Hauser, "Polysaccharides of Blastomyces Dermatitidis."
41. For a list of these see Bayard Carter and C. P. Jones, "A Study of the Vaginal Flora in the Normal Female," pp. 302–03.
42. Interview with Dr. F. Bayard Carter, 5 March 1969.
43. Carter and Jones, pp. 298–304; Bayard Carter, "A Bacteriologic Study of Pyometra."
44. Claudius P. Jones and Donald S. Martin, "Identification of Yeastlike

Organisms Isolated from the Vaginal Tracts of Pregnant and Nonpregnant Women"; Donald S. Martin, Claudius P. Jones, K. F. Yao and L. E. Lee, Jr., "A Practical Classification of the Monilias," pp. 99–122; Donald S. Martin and Claudius P. Jones, "Further Studies on the Practical Classification of the Monilias."

45. Walter A. Mickle and Claudius P. Jones, "Disassociation of Candida Albicans by Lithium Chloride and Immune Serum."

46. Bayard Carter, Claudius P. Jones, R. A. Ross, and Walter L. Thomas, "Vulvovaginal Mycoses in Pregnancy."

47. For a short history and bibliography of these discoveries up to the point that Hamblen began his work see, Edward C. Hamblen, "Clinical Experience with Follicular and Hypophyseal Hormones," pp. 184, 192–94.

48. James Harvey Young, *The Medical Messiahs*, pp. 149–50; Gerald Carson, *The Roguish World of Dr. Brinkley*, p. 166.

49. "Injectable Ovarian Preparations Omitted from N.N.R."

50. Young, p. 150.

51. Dr. George Johnson (Wilmington, N.C.) quoted in *Transactions* (1932) : 440.

52. E. C. Hamblen, "Human Ovarian Responses to Extracts of Pregnancy Urine—A Preliminay Report," pp. 286–87.

53. E. C. Hamblen, "Clinical Experience with Follicular and Hypophyseal Hormones," pp. 184–94; E. C. Hamblen, "Clinical Experience with Follicular and Anterior Pituitary Sex Hormones: A Study of the Results of Treatments in 120 Patients," pp. 464–73.

54. Interview with Dr. Robert A. Ross, 12 March 1969.

55. E. C. Hamblen, *Endocrine Gynecology*, p. 97.

56. E. C. Hamblen, "Clinical Correlates of Functional Uterine Bleeding"; Hamblen, *Endocrine Gynecology*, p. 210ff.

57. E. C. Hamblen, "Results of Preoperative Administration of an Extract of Pregnancy Urine"; E. C. Hamblen and R. A. Ross, "A Study of Ovaries Following Preoperative Administration of an Extract of Pregnancy Urine."

58. See, for example, E. C. Hamblen, "Present Concepts of Female Sex Hormones and Their Clinical Importance"; E. C. Hamblen, "Clinical Importance of the Female Sex Hormones," pp. 435–37.

59. E. C. Hamblen, "Therapeutic Use of the Sex Sterols in Functional Meno-Metrorragia," pp. 15–17, 27–28.

60. Hamblen, "Clinical Correlates of Functional Uterine Bleeding," pp. 308–19; Hamblen, *Endocrine Gynecology*.

61. E. C. Hamblen, et al., "Some Clinical Observations on the Metabolism and Utilization of Crystalline Progesterone"; E. C. Hamblen, W. K. Cuyler, and D. V. Hirst, "Studies of Urinary Excretions of Pregnandial-Complex by Males."

62. Interview with Dr. Robert A. Ross, 12 March 1969.

63. E. C. Hamblen, et al., "Studies of the Metabolism of Androgens in Women"; E. C. Hamblen, W. Kenneth Cuyler, and Margaret Baptist, "Urinary Androgens and Uterine Bleeding."

64. E. C. Hamblen, W. K. Cuyler, and Margaret Baptist, "Urinary Excretion of 17-Ketosteroids in Ovarian Failure."

65. E. C. Hamblen, "Rationale of Androgenic Therapy in Gynecology."

66. E. C. Hamblen, *Facts for Childless Couples,* pp. 3–13, 50–75.

67. E. C. Hamblen, et al., "Endocrine Therapy of Functional Meno-Metror-ragia and Ovarian Sterility."

68. Deryl Hart, "Sterilization of the Air in the Operating Room by Special Bactericidal Radiant Energy," p. 45; Deryl Hart, "Sterilization of the Air in the Operating Room by Bactericidal Radiant Energy," p. 770.

69. Deryl Hart and Samuel E. Upchurch, " 'Unexplained' Infections in Clean Operative Wounds," p. 939.

70. Deryl Hart, "Operation Room Infections."

71. Deryl Hart and Clarence E. Gardner, Jr., "Sterilization of the Air in the Operative Region with Bactericidal Radiant Energy," pp. 376–79.

72. Deryl Hart and Herman M. Schiebel, "Role of the Respiratory Tract in the Contamination of Air"; Hart and Upchurch, " 'Unexplained' Infections in Clean Operative Wounds," p. 939.

73. Hart, "Sterilization of the Air in the Operating Room by Special Bactericidal Radiant Energy" p. 45.

74. D. T. Smith, "Discussion," *Journal of Thoracic Surgery,* 7 (June 1938) : 535; Austin L. Joyner and David T. Smith, "Acute Staphylococcus Osteomyelitis."

75. Hart, "Operation Room Infections," pp. 879–82.

76. Hart and Upchurch, " 'Unexplained' Infections in Clean Operative Wounds," p. 947; Hart and Schiebel, p. 790; Hart and Gardner, p. 386.

77. Deryl Hart, "The Importance of Air-Borne Pathogenic Bacteria in the Operating Room," in F. R. Moulton, ed., *Aerobiology,* p. 188.

78. Hart, "Sterilization of the Air in the Operating Room by Special Bactericidal Radiant Energy," p. 53.

79. Hart, "Operating Room Infections," pp. 883–85; D. Gordon Sharp, "A Quantitative Method of Determining the Lethal Effect of Ultraviolet Light on Bacteria Suspended in Air." For subsequent variation see Hart, "The Importance of Air-Borne Pathogenic Bacteria . . . ," pp. 189–90.

80. Deryl Hart, John W. Devine, and D. W. Martin, "Bactericidal and Fungicidal Effect of Ultraviolet Radiation."

81. Hart, "Sterilization of the Air in the Operating Room by Special Bactericidal Radiant Energy," p. 59.

82. Deryl Hart and Paul W. Sanger, "Effect on Wound Healing of Bactericidal Ultraviolet Radiation from a Special Unit."

83. Hart, "Sterilization of the Air in the Operating Room by Special Bactericidal Radiant Energy," pp. 59–60.

84. Deryl Hart, "Sterilization of the Air in the Operating Room with Bactericidal Radiation," *Archives of Surgery,* 41 (Aug. 1940) : 334.

85. Deryl Hart, "Control of Air-Borne Pathogenic Bacteria by Bactericidal Radiant Energy."

86. Hart, "Operating Room Infections," p. 889.

87. Deryl Hart, "Sterilization of the Air in the Operating Room with Bactericidal Radiation," *Journal of Thoracic Surgery,* 7 (June 1938) : 525–27.

88. Deryl Hart and S. E. Upchurch, "Postoperative Temperature Reactions."

89. Hart, "Sterilization of the Air in the Operating Room with Bactericidal Radiation," pp. 526–32; Deryl Hart, "Sterilization of the Air in the Operat-

ing Room by Bactericidal Radiant Energy: Results in Over Eight Hundred Operations," pp. 956–64.

90. *The Evening Sun* (Baltimore, Maryland), 18 Nov. 1936.
91. Deryl Hart, "Pathogenic Bacteria in the Air of Operating Rooms."
92. Wilburt C. Davison, "Deryl Hart: Professor of Surgery, Duke University School of Medicine," (20 Oct. 1955), Clarence E. Gardner, Jr., Papers.
93. C. J. Kraisal, C. J. Cimiotte, and F. L. Meleney, "Considerations in the Use of Ultraviolet Radiation in Operating Rooms," pp. 177–78; Dr. W. Walters, "Discussion," p. 308; Hart, "Sterilization of the Air in the Operating Room with Bactericidal Radiation," pp. 341–45.
94. Dr. Isadore Cohn, "Discussion"; Deryl Hart, "Discussion."
95. Hart and Upchurch, " 'Unexplained' Infections in Clean Operative Wounds," pp. 938–56.
96. Clement Monroe quoted in Hart and Upchurch, " 'Unexplained' Infections in Clean Operative Wounds," pp. 947–49.
97. R. H. Overholt and R. H. Betts, "A Comparative Report on Infection of Thoracoplasty Wounds: Experiences with Ultraviolet Irradiation of Operating Room Air."
98. Hart and Upchurch, " 'Unexplained' Infections in Clean Operative Wounds," p. 945. This article contains charts summarizing the complete experience with ultraviolet bactericidal energy on each surgical service at Duke through 1940.
99. Deryl Hart, "Is Sterilization of the Air by the Use of Ultraviolet Radiation of Benefit?" For Hart's description of the place of this procedure in the total operating room sterile procedures, see Deryl Hart, "Minimizing the Contamination of Operative Wounds"; Dr. Reginald H. Jackson, "Discussion."
100. Interviews with Dr. Frederick Bernheim and Dr. Mary L. C. Bernheim, 26 Feb. 1969.
101. Frederick Bernheim, "Relation Between the Action of Histamin, Atropin, Adrenalin, and Heavy Metals on the Intestine."
102. See, for example, Frederick Bernheim, "The Interaction of Histamin and Nicotine on the Intestine"; Frederick Bernheim, "Action of Acetylcholine on the Intestine."
103. Frederick Bernheim, *The Interaction of Drugs and Cell Catalysts,* p. ii; interviews with Dr. Frederick Bernheim and Dr. Mary L. C. Bernheim, 26 Feb. 1969.
104. Frederick Bernheim, "The Effect of Alloxan on the Oxidation of Alcohol by Various Tissues."
105. Frederick Bernheim and Mary L. C. Bernheim, "The Hydrolysis of Homatropins and Atropine by Various Tissues."
106. Frederick Bernheim, "The Action of Papain and Trypsin on Certain Dehydrogenases."
107. Frederick Bernheim, *Interaction of Drugs and Cell Catalysts.*
108. Frederick Bernheim, "The Effect of Salicylate on the Oxygen Uptake of the Tubercle Bacillus."
109. Interviews with Dr. Frederick Bernheim and Dr. Mary L. C. Bernheim, 26 Feb. 1969.

110. Jorgen Lehmann, "Para-Aminosalicylic Acid in the Treatment of Tuberculosis."
111. *Report of the Committee on the School of Medicine and Hospital to the Board of Trustees of Duke University* (5 June 1937), Office of the Secretary, Duke University.
112. Interview with Dr. J. Deryl Hart, 26 Feb. 1969.
113. Interview with Dr. Joseph W. Beard, 25 Feb. 1969.
114. For Beard's work at the Rockefeller Institute, see Peyton Rouse, "Viruses and Tumors," in Thomas M. Rivers, et al., *Virus Diseases*, pp. 147–70, and George W. Corner, *A History of the Rockefeller Institute*, pp. 185, 213, 226, 394.
115. J. W. Beard and Ralph W. G. Wyckoff, "The Isolation of a Homogenous Heavy Protein from Virus-Induced Rabbit Papillomas."
116. Interview with Dr. Joseph W. Beard, 25 Feb. 1969.
117. J. W. Beard, Harold Finkelstein, and W. C. Sealy, "The Ultracentrifugal Concentration of the Immunizing Principle from Tissues Diseased with Equine Encephalomyelitis."
118. Ralph W. C. Wyckoff, "Ultracentrifugal Concentration of a Homogenous Heavy Component from Tissues Diseased with Equine Encephalomyelitis."
119. Interview with Dr. J. W. Beard, 25 Feb. 1969.
120. Ibid.
121. J. W. Beard, et al., "Immunization against Equine Encephalomyelitis with Chick Embryo Vaccines."
122. Interview with Dr. J. W. Beard, 25 Feb. 1969.
123. LeRoy D. Fothergill, et al., "Human Encephalitis Caused by the Virus of the Eastern Variety of Equine Encephalomyelitis."
124. J. W. Beard, Dorothy Beard, and Harold Finkelstein, "Human Vaccination against Equine Encephalomyelitis Virus with Formolized Chick Embryo Vaccine."
125. J. W. Beard, Dorothy Beard, and Harold Finkelstein, "Vaccination of Man Against the Virus of Equine Encephalomyelitis (Eastern and Western Strains)."
126. Interview with Dr. J. W. Beard, 25 Feb. 1969.
127. For a discussion of this point, see *Federal Support of Basic Research in Institutions of Higher Learning*, pp. 20–22.

Chapter 8: Modernizing Medical Care: Cooperation with The Duke Endowment

1. The Duke Indenture, pp. 16–17, 25, 50–51.
2. *The Duke Endowment: Annual Report of the Hospital Section* (1925), pp. 28, 33–34, 144–45. Hereinafter cited as DEHS. Watson S. Rankin, "Address to the Durham Alumni Association," 11 Dec. 1936, Duke Endowment Papers.
3. DEHS (1927), pp. 92–106; (1929), pp. 56–80.
4. Rankin to Charles E. Holyes, 16 April 1929, Duke Endowment Papers.

5. DEHS (1928), pp. 160–62; (1931), pp. 80–81.
6. "Student Nurses Will Be College Girls at Duke University."
7. *Bulletin of Duke University*, 2, no. 1 (Jan. 1930): 18–19; 3, no. 6 (June 1931): 363–64.
8. School of Nursing and Education Committee Minutes, 29 March 1938, Duke University School of Nursing Papers.
9. W. C. Davison, Memo, "Nursing Education," 1942, Davison Papers.
10. A breakdown of the hours spent in each phase of the program for the years 1933 and 1934 is contained in an undated memo among the Davison Papers. See also "North Carolina Board of Nurse Examiners: Quarterly Reports of Duke Hospital," Annual Reports, 1934, 1935, 1936, 1937, Duke University School of Nursing Papers.
11. "School of Nursing Faculty Minutes," 11 Oct. 1939, Duke University School of Nursing Papers.
12. F. V. Altvater to the Members of the Nursing Committee, 22 Aug. 1940, Davison Papers.
13. Lucile Petry to W. C. Davison, 13 June 1939, Davison Papers.
14. *Bulletin of Duke University*, 13, no. 5C (April 1941): 92.
15. *Bulletin of Duke University*, 13, no. 3 (Feb. 1941): 20–24.
16. Richard H. Shryock, *The History of Nursing*, p. 310.
17. Agnes Gelenas, *Nursing and Nursing Education*, pp. 36–54.
18. Association of Collegiate Schools of Nursing, "Standards of Membership for Schools Offering a Basic Professional Curriculum in Nursing Leading to a Degree," 1937, Flowers Papers.
19. *Bulletin of Duke University*, 8, no. 2A (Feb. 1936): 21; 13, no. 5C (April 1941): 92.
20. Altvater to the Members of the Nursing Committee, 22 Aug. 1940, Davison Papers.
21. W. C. Davison to Stander, 10 Jan. 1941, Davison Papers.
22. Nursing Committee, Duke Hospital, undated report, Forbus Papers.
23. Undated memo, "The Nursing Department Problem at Duke Hospital," Davison Papers; interview with W. C. Davison by F. W. Rounds, May 1964.
24. Dorothy W. Beard, undated report, Davison Papers.
25. M. I. Pinkerton, undated report, Davison Papers.
26. School of Nursing Faculty Minutes, 7 Jan. 1941, Duke University School of Nursing Papers.
27. Abstract from Minutes of Executive Committee, 18 Nov. 1940; Sister M. Olivia Gowan to M. I. Pinkerton, 24 March 1941, Davison Papers.
28. Mrs. J. H. Martin to Dr. Clyde Brooks, 27 June 1930, Department of Dietetics Papers; "Hospital Courses for Student Dietitians Approved by the American Dietetic Association."
29. Mary I. Barber, ed., *History of the American Dietetic Association*, pp. 134–35.
30. Mrs. J. H. Martin to Dr. Clyde Brooks, 27 June 1930, Department of Dietetics Papers.
31. *Bulletin of Duke University*, 8, no. 1 (Jan. 1936): 29.
32. Transcripts showing the detail of the program of study are filed in the offices of the Department of Dietetics, Duke University Hospital. See also

"Hospital Courses for Student Dietitians Approved by the American Dietetic Association, 1932–1933," p. 230.

33. Davison, *The First Twenty Years*, p. 47.

34. David T. Smith, "To whom it may concern," 7 April 1943, Medical Technology School Papers.

35. "Record of Practical Training and Work Completed at Duke University Hospital," Medical Technology School Papers.

36. Interview with Dr. David T. Smith, 14 April 1969.

37. Transcripts showing the origin of the students are filed in the offices of the Medical Technology School, Veterans Administration Hospital, Durham, N.C.; *Bulletin of Duke University*, 13, no. 3 (April 1941) : 120.

38. F. Ross Porter and W. C. Davison, "The Role, Problems, Responsibilities and Training of a Hospital Administrator."

39. Michael M. Davis, *Hospital Administration: A Career*, pp. ii, 33–53.

40. Porter and Davison; interview with F. Vernon Altvater, 21 Dec. 1968.

41. Duke University Hospital Administration Alumni List (July 1967), Department of Hospital Administration Papers; Rankin to Davison, 26 Oct. 1937, Duke Endowment Papers.

42. *Bulletin of Duke University*, 13, no. 3 (Feb. 1931) : 20–24.

43. *Bulletin of Duke University*, 11, no. 3 (March 1939) : 101; 13, no. 5C (April 1941) : 113.

44. Watson S. Rankin, "The Duke Endowment" (1 June 1939), Duke Endowment Papers.

45. Rankin to Forbus, 14 March 1932; 27 May 1933, Forbus Papers; Rankin to Davison, 24 March 1933, Davison Papers.

46. Gunnar Myrdal, *An American Dilemma*, p. 323.

47. Rankin to Davison, 25 May 1933; George P. Harris, Memo, "Lincoln Hospital," 10 May 1933, "Lincoln Hospital, Durham, N.C., Comparative Statement, 1932 and 1933," Duke Endowment Papers; Dr. Foy Roberson, M. E. Newsom, and C. C. Spaulding to the Trustees of Lincoln Hospital, 17 April 1934, Flowers Papers.

48. Rankin to M. M. Davis, 1 March 1934, Duke Endowment Papers.

49. Rankin to S. L. Warren, 6 July 1933, Flowers Papers.

50. Davison to Rankin, 21 Feb. 1934, Duke Endowment Papers.

51. James E. Shephard to Rankin, 31 March 1934, Duke Endowment Papers.

52. Davison to Rankin, 21 Feb. 1934, Duke Endowment Papers.

53. Rankin to Davison, 23 Feb. 1934, Duke Endowment Papers.

54. Davison to Dr. Warren, 6 March 1934, Duke Endowment Papers; Dr. Foy Roberson, M. E. Newsom, and C. C. Spaulding to The Trustees of Lincoln Hospital, 17 April 1934, Flowers Papers.

55. James E. Shephard to Rankin, 31 March 1934; M. E. Newsom to Davison, 20 April 1934, Duke Endowment Papers.

56. Davison to Rankin, 4 April 1934, Duke Endowment Papers.

57. Rankin to Davison, 28 Feb. 1934, Davison Papers.

58. N. J. Blackwood to Davison, 9 April 1934, Davison Papers.

59. M. E. Newsom to Davison, 20 April 1934; James C. Shephard to Rankin, 20 April 1934; memo, "Lincoln Hospital," undated, Duke Endowment Papers; C. Rufus Rorem to Davison, 4 June 1934, Davison Papers.

60. Interview with Dr. Robert A. Ross, 12 March 1969.

61. George P. Harris, Memorandum, "Lincoln Hospital," 19 Nov. 1934, Duke Endowment Papers.
62. The Duke Endowment, File of Resolutions, Lincoln Hospital, Durham, N.C., 25 June 1935, 26 Sept. 1936, Duke Endowment Papers.
63. A. D. K., Memorandum, "Lincoln Hospital," 22 Sept. 1936, Duke Endowment Papers.
64. Interview with Dr. Robert A. Ross, 12 March 1969.
65. W. S. Rankin, Memo, "In re Central Pathological Service for Assisted Hospitals," 25 April 1933, Duke Endowment Papers.
66. Forbus to Rankin, 30 Nov. 1931, Forbus Papers.
67. Forbus to Rankin, 24 Oct. 1932, Forbus Papers.
68. W. D. Forbus to W. C. Tate, 18 July 1933, Forbus Papers.
69. W. D. Forbus to H. L. Johnson, Sept. 1933, Forbus Papers.
70. Forbus to Rankin, 25 March 1933, Duke Endowment Papers.
71. Rankin to Forbus, 29 Oct. 1932, Forbus Papers.
72. Forbus to Rankin, 25 March 1933, Forbus Papers.
73. W. D. Forbus to Miss Sallie E. Lineberry, 29 April 1933, Forbus Papers.
74. Forbus to Rankin, 21 July 1933, Forbus Papers.
75. R. N. Harden to Forbus, 2 June 1933; J. L. Reeves to Forbus, 19 July 1933, Forbus Papers.
76. R. N. Harden to Forbus, 2 June 1933, Forbus Papers.
77. W. D. Forbus, "Report of the Department of Pathology," 18 Sept. 1933, Forbus Papers.
78. Forbus to Horace M. Baker, 16 Feb. 1933, Forbus Papers; Alex H. Sands, Jr., to Rankin, 30 March 1933, Duke Endowment Papers.
79. Forbus to Miss Sallie E. Lineberry, 2 May 1935, Forbus Papers.
80. Interview with W. D. Forbus, 8 April 1969.
81. DEHS (1925), pp. 38–41.
82. *Bulletin of Duke University*, 3, no. 6 (1931), 333. Davison, "Rural General Practice in Groups," pp. 180–89.
83. Dr. L. V. Grady quoted in *Durham Morning Herald*, 20 May 1931, p. 1.
84. *Durham Morning Herald*, 15 Oct. 1936, sec. 2, p. 8.
85. Programs from the first six symposia are included among the Hanes Papers.
86. *Durham Morning Herald*, 5 Nov. 1937, p. 8.
87. *Durham Herald-Sun*, 15 Oct. 1939, p. 4.
88. "Supplement and Changes to the Program of Post Graduate Course in Fractures, 12–13 Oct. 1934," Hanes Papers.
89. Rankin to Davison, 12 Dec. 1935, North Carolina Blue Cross-Blue Shield Papers.
90. *Durham Morning Herald*, 1 Nov. 1940, sec. 2, p. 3.
91. "Programme of Post Graduate Course in Gastrointestinal Diseases," 31 Oct.– 2 Nov. 1935, Hanes Papers.
92. See the programs for the symposia of 1937–1939, Hanes Papers; *Durham Morning Herald*, 1 Nov. 1940, sec. 2, p. 3.
93. W. D. Forbus, "Southern Pathological Conference Protocol," 1933, Forbus Papers.
94. *Durham Morning Herald*, 2 Aug. 1939, p. 1; 4 Aug. 1939, sec. 2, p. 8; 5 Aug. 1939, p. 12.

95. A. D. R., Memorandum, "Lincoln Hospital," 22 Sept. 1936, Duke Endowment Papers.

96. George P. Harris to William M. Rich, 14 Oct. 1940; 2 Nov. 1940, Duke Endowment Papers.

97. DEHS (1939), p. 34.

98. Watson S. Rankin, "The Duke Endowment," 1 June 1939, Duke Endowment Papers.

99. *The Duke Endowment Year Book*, no. 9 (1940), pp. 14–19; DEHS (1934), p. 24; (1939), pp. 7–9.

100. DEHS (1939), pp. 10–11.

101. M. Virginia Dwyer, ed., *American Medical Directory, 1958*, p. 12.

102. *Bulletin of Duke University*, 13, no. 5C (April, 1941), 100–01.

103. Michael M. Davis, "Who Finances Construction?" in Arthur C. Bachmeyer, ed., *The Hospital in Modern Society*, p. 62.

104. Franklin D. Roosevelt, "Address to Advisory Council of the Committee on Economic Security on the Problems of Economic and Social Security, November 14, 1934," in Samuel I. Rosenman, ed., *The Public Papers and Addresses of Franklin D. Roosevelt*, 3: 452–55. Hereinafter cited as Rosenman.

105. Rosenman, 4: 326–27.

106. W. C. Davison, "The Duke Endowment," undated typescript, Davison Papers.

107. Interdepartmental Committee to Coordinate Health and Welfare Activities, *A National Health Program: Report of the Technical Committee on Medical Care, 1938*, pp. 1–4.

108. U.S., Congress, Senate, Committee on Education and Labor, *Hearings*, S.3230, 76th Cong., 3rd sess., 1940.

109. U.S., Congress, Senate, Committee on Education and Labor, *Hearings*, S.191, 79th Cong., 1st sess., 1945, pp. 211, 285–87, 323–28.

110. Ibid., p. 286.

Chapter 9: The Regional Medical Center: End of an Era, 1940–1941

1. Davison, *The First Twenty Years*, p. 8.

2. *A Study of Mental Health in North Carolina*, pp. 313–17; *Bulletin of Duke University*, 6, no. 1 (Jan. 1934): 35–36.

3. Raymond S. Crispell, "Report on the First Year of a Full-Time Division of Neuropsychiatry."

4. *A Study of Mental Health in North Carolina*, pp. vi, xvi, 167–83, 226, 357, 368.

5. Ibid., p. vi.

6. Clark R. Cahow, "The History of the North Carolina Mental Hospitals, 1848–1960" (unpublished Ph.D. dissertation, Dept. of History, Duke University, 1967), pp. 70–72. I am indebted to Mr. Cahow for his aid in establishing the sequence of these events.

7. W. C. Davison to Alan Gregg, 12 April 1938, Davison Papers.

8. "Minutes, Duke Trustees," 10 Dec. 1938, 1 Feb. 1938, 1 March 1939.
9. *The Rockefeller Foundation Annual Report for 1940*, pp. 144–45.
10. For an insight on the critical importance of the dean in conducting a successful medical school during this decade see Herman G. Weiskotten, et al., *Medical Education in the United States, 1934–1939*, pp. 40–46.
11. Davison, "The First Ten Years . . . ," pp. 2–3.
12. Clarence Poe, ed., *Hospital and Medical Care for All Our People*, pp. 18–19.
13. Poe, pp. 1–4.
14. Coy C. Carpenter, "A History of Wake Forest University in the Field of Medical Education with Personal Reminiscences by the Author," unpublished manuscript, 1968, pp. 42–43.
15. William deB. MacNider to Davison, 19 Jan. 1937; Davison to Watson S. Rankin, 19 Jan. 1937, Davison Papers.
16. Carpenter, pp. 44–45.
17. George Washington Paschal, *History of Wake Forest College*, 3: 433–34.
18. Raleigh *News and Observer*, 14 Nov. 1929.
19. Carpenter, p. 42.
20. William DeB. MacNider to Davison, 2 Nov. 1935, Davison Papers.
21. Raleigh *News and Observer*, 1 Oct. 1935; 2 Oct. 1935.
22. Carpenter, pp. 46–49.
23. Wilburt C. Davison, "Greetings from Duke University School of Medicine at the Laying of the Cornerstone of the Bowman Gray School of Medicine of Wake Forest College," 16 April 1941, Davison Papers.
24. Davison, *The First Twenty Years*, p. 72.
25. War Department, "General Hospital" (T/O 8-550) (Washington, 1 April 1942), pp. 2–3. Copy in Elbert L. Persons, Jr., Papers.
26. Wilburt C. Davison, memo, "Information obtained at War Dept. 10/30/40," Forbus Papers.
27. Davison, *The First Twenty Years*, p. 81.
28. William D. Cutter to Wilburt C. Davison, 31 July 1940, copy in Forbus Papers.
29. James O. Kelly, "Shall Medical Defense Be Depleted?"
30. Lewis B. Hershey to All State Directors, 21 April 1941, Forbus Papers.
31. Selective Service Board #334 to Deryl Hart, 20 Feb. 1941, Forbus Papers.
32. Several drafts to these letters are among the Forbus Papers.
33. Frederic M. Hanes, "Dedicatory Talk."
34. Memo, "Report of the Activities of the Duke Council for American Defense," undated, Forbus Papers; *Durham Morning Herald*, 12 Nov. 1940; 22 Dec. 1940; 30 Jan. 1941; 6 Nov. 1941.
35. *Durham Morning Herald*, 14 Oct. 1941.
36. *Durham Morning Herald*, 17–18 Oct. 1941.
37. Elbert L. Persons to 65th General Hospital, 13 Oct. 1941, Elbert L. Persons Papers.
38. Davison, *The First Twenty Years*, p. 73.
39. *Durham Morning Herald*, 18 Oct. 1941.

Works Cited

Articles

Altvater, F. Vernon. "A Flat Rate Plan Designed to Help Both Hospital and Patient." *The Modern Hospital* 41 (Aug. 1933) : 71–75.
———. "Flat Rates for 4½ Years." *Modern Hospital* 49 (Dec. 1937) : 47–48.
———. "Theory and Application of Inclusive or Flat Rate Plans." *Hospitals* 14 (Oct. 1940) : 61–66.
Baker, Roger D. "Case Method and Clerkship in Teaching Pathology." *Journal of the Association of American Medical Colleges* 12 (May 1937) : 165–72.
Bass, C. C. "Demands on the Medical Practitioner in the South During One Year." *Bulletin of the Association of American Medical Colleges* 3 (1928) : 305–11.
Beard, J. W., Dorothy Beard and Harold Finkelstein. "Human Vaccination against Equine Encephalomyelitis Virus with Formolized Chick Embroyo Vaccine." *Science* 90 (1 Sept. 1939) : 215–16.
———, et al. "Immunization Against Equine Encephalomyelitis with Chick Embryo Vaccines." *Science* 87 (27 May 1938) : 490.
——— and Ralph W. G. Wyckoff. "The Isolation of a Homogenous Heavy Protein from Virus-Induced Rabbit Papillomas." *Science* 85 (19 Feb. 1937) : 201–02.
———, Harold Finkelstein and W. C. Sealy. "The Ultracentrifugal Concentration of the Immunizing Principle from Tissues Diseased with Equine Encephalomyelitis." *Science* 87 (28 Jan. 1938) : 89–90.
———, Dorothy Beard and Harold Finkelstein. "Vaccination of Man Against the Virus of Equine Encephalomyelitis (Eastern and Western Strains)." *Journal of Immunology* 38 (Feb. 1940) : 117–36.
Bernheim, Frederick. "Action of Acetylcholine on the Intestine." *American Journal of Physiology* 104 (May 1933) : 433–37.
———. "The Action of Papain and Trypsin on Certain Dehydrogenases." *Journal of Biological Chemistry* 133 (March 1940) : 141–44.
———. "The Effect of Alloxan on the Oxidation of Alcohol by Various Tissues." *Journal of Biological Chemistry* 123 (May 1938) : 741–49.
———. "The Effect of Salicylate on the Oxygen Uptake of the Tubercle Bacillus." *Science* 92 (30 Aug. 1940), 204.
——— and Mary L. C. Bernheim. "The Hydrolysis of Homatropins and Atropine by Various Tissues." *Journal of Pharmacology and Experimental Therapeutics* 64 (Oct. 1938) : 209–16.
———. "The Interaction of Histamin and Nicotine on the Intestine." *Journal of Pharmacology and Experimental Therapeutics* 48 (May 1933) : 67–72.
———. "Relation Between the Action of Histamin, Atropin, Adrenalin, and Heavy Metals on the Intestine." *Journal of Pharmacology and Experimental Therapeutics* 42 (Aug. 1931) : 441–54.
Blue, Willis B., and Wilburt C. Davison. "The Evolution of Infant Feeding and the Advantages and Disadvantages of Soured Milk Mixtures." *Postgraduate Medicine* 20 (July 1956), 41–48.

Carter, Bayard. "A Bacteriologic Study of Pyometra." *American Journal of Obstetrics and Gynecology* 44 (Dec. 1942) : 1074–90.

——— and C. P. Jones. "A Study of the Vaginal Flora in the Normal Female." *Southern Medical Journal* 30 (March 1937) : 298–304.

———, Claudius P. Jones, R. A. Ross and Walter L. Thomas. "Vulvovaginal Mycoses in Pregnancy." *American Journal of Obstetrics and Gynecology* 39 (Feb. 1940) : 213–26.

Cason, T. Z. "The Progress of Medical Research in the South." *Annals of Internal Medicine* 2 (Oct. 1928) : 309–15.

Chase, Harry W. "Medical Education." *Southern Medicine and Surgery* 76 (March 1924) : 116–19.

Cohn, Isadore. "Discussion." *Annals of Surgery* 110 (Aug. 1939) : 309.

Council on Medical Education and Hospitals of the American Medical Association. "Medical Education in the United States and Canada." *Journal of the American Medical Association* 115 (31 Aug. 1940) : 685–701.

Crispell, Raymond S. "Report on the First Year of a Full-Time Division of Neuropsychiatry." *Southern Medicine and Surgery* 97 (Jan. 1935) : 1–4.

Daun, W. S. "Nicotinic Acid and Vitamin B₂." *Science* 86 (31 Dec. 1937) : 616–17.

Davis, Graham L. "Hospital Insurance Why Not?". *Hospital Management* 31 (Feb. 1931) : 54–58.

Davis, Michael M. "Problems of Health Service for Negroes." *Journal of Negro Education,* 6 (July 1937) : 438–49.

Davison, Wilburt C. "The Birth of Blue Cross." *Virginia Medical Monthly* 91 (Nov. 1964) : 481–82.

———. "Changes in Medical Education and Patient Care." *The Journal of the Florida Medical Association* 41 (Sept. 1954) : 173–84.

———. "The Diagnosis of Enteric Fever (Typhoid and Paratyphoid A and B) by Agglutination Tests." *Journal of the American Medical Association* 46 (22 April 1916) : 1297–1300.

———. "The Duke Private Diagnostic Clinic." *Journal of Medical Education* 31 (July 1956) : 482–84.

———. "The Duke University School of Medicine." *Transactions of the Medical Society of the State of North Carolina* 74 (1927) : 35–39.

———. "The First Ten Years of the Duke University School of Medicine and Hospital." *North Carolina Medical Journal* 2 (Oct. 1941) : 527–32.

———. "The Future of American Pediatrics." *The Journal of Pediatrics* 14 (June 1939) : 810–14.

———. "The Future of Medical Education." *Journal of the Association of American Medical Colleges* 21 (July 1946) : 223–35.

———. "John Howland." *Journal of Pediatrics* 46 (April 1955) : 473–86.

———. "Liberalizing the Curriculum." *Southern Medical Journal* 21 (Dec. 1928) : 983–87.

———. "An M.D. Degree Five Years After High School." *Journal of the American Medical Association* 90 (2 June 1928) : 1812–16.

———. "Opportunities in the Practice of Medicine." *Journal of the American Medical Association* 115 (21 Dec. 1940) : 2227–32.

———. "Pediatric Diagnosis." *The Journal of Pediatrics* 9 (Aug. 1936) : 209–14.

———. "Qualities Which a Medical Student and Physician Should Have or

Develop." *Journal of the Association of American Medical Colleges* 16 (Sept. 1941) : 278–81.

———. "Rural General Practice in Groups." *Journal of the Association of American Medical Colleges* 73 (May 1948) : 180–89.

———. "The Selection of Medical Students." *Southern Medical Journal* 20 (Dec. 1927) : 955–60.

———. "The Significance of Present Entrance Requirements." *Journal of the American Medical Association* 96 (25 April 1931) : 1367–69.

———. "Sir William Osler, Reminiscences." *Archives of Internal Medicine* 84 (July 1949) : 110–28.

———. "The 1915 Serbian Typhus Epidemic." *North Carolina Medical Journal* 5 (July 1944) , 282–85.

———. "Two Additional Years in College Versus Two More Years in Hospital." *Southern Medical Journal* 23 (Sept. 1930) : 851–55.

"Dedication of the Duke University School of Medicine and Hospital." *Southern Medical Journal* 26 (Dec. 1931) : 1099–124.

"Duke Hospital Clinico-Pathological Conference, November 8, 1939." *North Carolina Medical Journal* 1 (May 1940) : 260–64.

Elvehjem, C. A., R. J. Madden, F. M. Strong and D. W. Woolley. "Relation of Nicotinic Acid and Nicotinic Amide to Canine Black Tongue." *Journal of the American Chemical Society* 59 (Sept. 1937) : 1767.

———, R. J. Madden, F. M. Strong and D. W. Woolley. "The Isolation and Identification of the Anti-Blacktongue Factor." *Journal of Biological Chemistry* 123 (March 1938) : 137–49.

Falk, I. S. "An Introduction to National Problems in Medical Care." *Law and Contemporary Problems* 6 (Autumn 1939) : 497–506.

Forbus, Wiley T., and John S. Bradway. "Medicolegal Investigation." *Southern Medical Journal* 26 (Sept. 1933) : 768–71.

Fothergill, LeRoy D., et al. "Human Encephalitis Caused by the Virus of the Eastern Variety of Equine Encephalomyelitis." *The New England Journal of Medicine* 219 (22 Sept. 1938) : 411.

Hamblen, E. C. "Clinical Correlates of Functional Uterine Bleeding." *The Southern Medical Journal* 32 (March 1939) : 308–19.

———. "Clinical Experience with Follicular and Anterior Pituitary Sex Hormones: A Study of the Results of Treatment in 120 Patients." *Virginia Medical Monthly* 59 (Nov. 1932) : 464–74.

———. "Clinical Experience with Follicular and Hypophyseal Hormones." *Endocrinology* 15 (May-June 1931) : 184–94.

———. "Clinical Importance of the Female Sex Hormones." *Transactions of the Medical Society of the State of North Carolina* 79 (1932) : 435–64.

———, et al. "Endocrine Therapy of Functional Meno-Metrorrhagia and Ovarian Sterility." *The Journal of Clinical Endocrinology* 1 (March 1941) : 211–27; (Sept. 1941) : 742–53.

———. "Human Ovarian Responses to Extracts of Pregnancy Urine—A Preliminary Report." *Virginia Medical Monthly* 60 (Aug. 1933) : 286–90.

———. "Present Concepts of Female Sex Hormones and Their Clinical Importance." *Virginia Medical Monthly* 58 (Nov. 1931) : 509–12.

———. "Rationale of Androgenic Therapy in Gynecology." *The Journal of Clinical Endocrinology* 1 (Feb. 1941) : 180–86.

————. "Results of Preoperative Administration of an Extract of Pregnancy Urine." *Endocrinology* 19 (March–April 1935) : 169–80.

————, et al. "Some Clinical Observations on the Metabolism and Utilization of Crystalline Progesterone." *Endocrinology* 25 (July 1939) : 13–16.

————, et al. "Studies of the Metabolism of Androgens in Women." *Endocrinology* 25 (Oct. 1939) : 491–508.

————, W. K. Cuyler and D. V. Hirst. "Studies of Urinary Excretions of Pregnandial-Complex by Males." *Endocrinology* 27 (Aug. 1940) : 169–71.

———— and R. A. Ross. "A Study of Ovaries Following Preoperative Administration of an Extract of Pregnancy Urine." *American Journal of Obstetrics and Gynecology* 31 (Jan. 1936) : 14–29.

————. "Therapeutic Use of the Sex Sterols in Functional Meno-Metrorrhagia." *Endocrinology* 24 (Jan. 1939) : 13–28.

————, W. Kenneth Cuyler and Margaret Baptist. "Urinary Androgens and Uterine Bleeding." *Endocrinology* 27 (July 1940) : 16–18.

————, W. Kenneth Cuyler and Margaret Baptist. "Urinary Excretion of 17–Ketosteroids in Ovarian Failure." *The Journal of Clinical Endocrinology* 1 (Sept. 1941) : 763–81.

Hanes, Frederic M. "Dedicatory Talk." *North Carolina Medical Journal* 2 (March 1941) : 146.

———— and Wilburt C. Davison. "Postgraduate Medical Education and Internships." *Journal of the Association of American Medical Colleges* 16 (Nov. 1941) : 371–74.

Hart, Deryl. "Control of Air-Borne Pathogenic Bacteria by Bactericidal Radiant Energy." *The Modern Hospital* 46 (June 1936) : 79–81.

————, John W. Devine and D. W. Martin. "Bactericidal and Fungicidal Effect of Ultraviolet Radiation." *Archives of Surgery* 38 (May 1939) : 806–15.

————. "Discussion." *Annals of Surgery* 110 (Aug. 1939) : 310.

———— and Paul W. Sanger. "Effect on Wound Healing of Bactericidal Ultraviolet Radiation from a Special Unit." *Archives of Surgery* 38 (May 1939) : 797–805.

————. "Is Sterilization of the Air by the Use of Ultraviolet Radiation of Benefit?" *International Abstracts of Surgery* 71 (Nov. 1940) : 420–22.

————. "Minimizing the Contamination of Operative Wounds." *Surgical Clinics of North America* 22 (April 1942) : 357–76.

————. "Operation Room Infections." *Archives of Surgery* 34 (May 1937) : 874–77.

————. "Pathogenic Bacteria in the Air of Operating Rooms." *Archives of Surgery* 37 (Oct. 1933) : 521–30.

———— and S. E. Upchurch. "Postoperative Temperature Reactions." *Annals of Surgery* 110 (Aug. 1939) : 291–306.

————. "The Responsibility of the Medical Profession to Medical Education." *Annals of Surgery* 145 (May 1957) : 599–623.

———— and Herman M. Schiebel. "Role of the Respiratory Tract in the Contamination of Air." *Archives of Surgery* 38 (April 1939) : 788–96.

————. "Sterilization of the Air in the Operating Room by Bactericidal Radiant Energy." *Surgery* 1 (May 1937) : 770–84.

————. "Sterilization of the Air in the Operating Room by Bactericidal Radiant Energy: Results in Over Eight Hundred Operations." *Archives of Surgery* 37 (Dec. 1938) : 156–72.

———. "Sterilization of the Air in the Operating Room by Special Bactericidal Radiant Energy." *Journal of Thoracic Surgery* 6 (Oct. 1936) : 45–81.

———. "Sterilization of the Air in the Operating Room with Bactericidal Radiation." *Archives of Surgery* 41 (Aug. 1940) : 334–350.

———. "Sterilization of the Air in the Operating Room with Bactericidal Radiation." *Journal of Thoracic Surgery* 7 (June 1938) : 525–35.

——— and Clarence E. Gardner, Jr. "Sterilization of the Air in the Operative Region with Bactericidal Radiant Energy." *Transactions of the Southern Surgical Association* 49 (1937) : 376–402.

——— and Samuel E. Upchurch. " 'Unexplained' Infections in Clean Operative Wounds." *Annals of Surgery* 114 (Nov. 1941) : 936–59.

Harvey, H. I., D. T. Smith, E. L. Persons and M. V. Burns, "The Effect of Various Fractions of Liver on Experimental Canine Blacktongue." *Journal of Nutrition* 16 (Aug. 1938) : 153–71.

Hill, John Sprunt. "Remarks on the History of Watts Hospital." *Southern Medicine and Surgery* 107 (May 1945) : 171–72.

Hils, R. G. "Prices, Business Activity and War." *Hospitals* 14 (Jan. 1940) : 96–98.

"Hospital Courses for Student Dietitians Approved by the American Dietetic Association." *Journal of the American Dietetic Association* 7 (June 1931) : 52–54.

"Hospital Courses for Student Dietitians Approved by the American Dietetic Association, 1932–1933." *Journal of the American Dietetic Association* 9 (Sept. 1933) : 226–32.

"Hospitalization Insurance." *Textile Bulletin* 54 (28 April 1938) : 14–15.

"Injectable Ovarian Preparations Omitted from N. N. R." *Journal of the American Medical Association* 98 (30 Jan. 1932) : 402.

Jackson, Reginald H. "Discussion." *Annals of Surgery* 110 (Aug. 1939) : 307–08.

Jones, Claudius P., and Donald S. Martin. "Identification of Yeastlike Organisms Isolated from the Vaginal Tracts of Pregnant and Nonpregnant Women." *American Journal of Obstetrics and Gynecology* 35 (Jan. 1938) : 98–106.

Joyner, Austin L., and David T. Smith. "Acute Staphylococcus Osteomyelitis." *Surgery, Gynecology and Obstetrics* 63 (July 1936) : 1–6.

Kelly, James O. "Shall Medical Defense Be Depleted?" *The Milwaukee Medical Times* 14 (March 1941) : 13–14.

Kraisal, C. J., C. J. Cimiette and F. L. Meleney. "Considerations in the Use of Ultraviolet Radiation in Operating Rooms." *Annals of Surgery* 111 (Feb. 1940) : 161–85.

Lassek, A. M. "The Role of the Southeastern Schools of Medicine in the National Distribution of Physicians." *Journal of the Association of American Medical Colleges* 19 (July 1944) : 217–23.

Lehmann, Jorgen. "Para-Aminosalicylic Acid in the Treatment of Tuberculosis." *The Lancet* 250 (5 Jan. 1946) : 15–16.

Margolis, G., L. H. Margolis and S. G. Smith. "The Cure of Experimental Blacktongue and Optimal and Minimal Doses of Nicotinic Acid." *Journal of Nutrition* 16 (Dec. 1938) : 541–48.

Margolis, L. H., G. Margolis and S. G. Smith. "Secondary Deficiency of Vitamin B_2 and Riboflavin in the Blacktongue Producing Diet." *Journal of Nutrition* 17 (Jan. 1939) : 63–76.

Martin, Donald S., and David T. Smith. "Blastomycosis: A Report of Thirteen New Cases." *American Review of Tuberculosis* 39 (April 1939) : 488–515.

────── and D. T. Smith. "Blastomycosis: A Review of the Literature." *American Review of Tuberculosis* 39 (March 1939) : 275–304.

────── and N. F. Conant. "A Comparative Study of Nineteen Strains of Blastomyces Dermatitidis Gilchrist and Stokes, 1898." *Journal of Bacteriology* 35 (Jan. 1938) : 38–39.

──────. "Complement-Fixation in Blastomycosis." *Journal of Infectious Diseases* 57 (Dec. 1935) : 291–95.

────── and Claudius P. Jones. "Further Studies on Practical Classification of the Monilias." *Journal of Bacteriology* 39 (May 1940) : 609–30.

──────, Claudius P. Jones, K. F. Yao and L. E. Lee, Jr. "A Practical Classification of the Monilias." *Journal of Bacteriology* 34 (July 1937) : 99–129.

Mason, Cleon C. "Are Hospital Costs Too High?" *North American Review* 228 (July 1929) : 57–64.

McLendon, William W. "Edenborough Medical College." *North Carolina Medical Journal* 19 (Oct. 1958) : 433–40.

"Medical Education in the United States and Canada." *Journal of the American Medical Association* 103 (25 Aug. 1934) , 565–80.

Mickle, Walter A., and Claudius P. Jones. "Disassociation of Candida Albicans by Lithium Chloride and Immune Serum." *Journal of Bacteriology* 39 (June 1940) : 633–47.

Overholt, R. H., and R. H. Betts. "A Comparative Report on Infection of Thoracoplasty Wounds: Experiences with Ultraviolet Irradiation of Operating Room Air." *Journal of Thoracic Surgery* 9 (June 1940) : 520–29.

Peck, Robert L., Donald S. Martin and Charles R. Hauser. "Polysaccharides of Blastomyses Dermatitidis." *Journal of Immunology* 38 (June 1940) : 449–55.

Perlzweig, W. A., E. D. Levy and H. Sarett. "On Quantitative Determination of Nicotinic Acid and its Derivatives in Urine." *Journal of Biological Chemistry* 138 (May 1940) : lxxiv–lxxv.

Porter, F. Ross, and Wilburt C. Davison. "The Role, Problems, Responsibilities and Training of a Hospital Administrator." *Journal of Medical Education* 29 (Feb. 1954) : 26–32.

Rankin, Watson S. "Economics of Medical Service." *American Journal of Public Health* 19 (April 1929) : 359–65.

Richardson, J. T. "The Origin and Development of Group Hospitalization in the United States, 1890–1940." *The University of Missouri Studies* 20, no. 3 (1945) : 9–101.

Ruffin, Julian M., E. L. Persons, H. I. Harvey and D. T. Smith. "Evidence for the Existence of Two Factors Necessary for the Successful Treatment of Pellagra or Experimental Canine Black Tongue." *Journal of Clinical Investigation* 16 (Aug. 1937) : 663.

────── and David T. Smith. "A Clinical Evaluation of the Potency of Various Extracts of Liver in the Treatment of Pellagra." *The Southern Medical Journal* 30 (Jan. 1937) , 4–14.

──────. "A New Method of Teaching Physical Diagnosis." *Journal of the Association of American Medical Colleges* 10 (Sept. 1935) : 292–94.

────── and David T. Smith. "Treatment of Pellagra with Special Reference to the Use of Nicotinic Acid." *The Southern Medical Journal* 32 (Jan. 1939) : 40–47.

Sharp, D. Gordon. "A Quantitative Method of Determining the Lethal Effect of Ultraviolet Light on Bacteria Suspended in Air." *Journal of Bacteriology* 35 (June 1938) : 589–99.

Smith, David T. "Discussion." *Southern Medicine and Surgery* 94 (March 1932) : 134.

———— and Donald S. Martin. "Blastomycosis." *National Tuberculosis Association Transactions* 32 (1936) : 70–72.

————. "Diagnosis and Treatment of Common Fungus Infections of the Lungs." *Transactions of the Twenty-Ninth Annual Meeting of the National Tuberculosis Association* 29 (1933) : 76–79.

————. "Diagnosis and Treatment of Fungus Infections in North Carolina." *Transactions of the Medical Society of the State of North Carolina* 80 (1933) : 598–602.

————. "Discussion." *Journal of Thoracic Surgery* 7 (June 1938) : 535.

———— and Julian M. Ruffin. "Effect of Sunlight on the Clinical Manifestations of Pellagra." *Archives of Internal Medicine* 59 (April 1937) : 631–45.

————, E. L. Persons and H. I. Harvey. "On the Identity of Goldberger and Underhill Types of Canine Blacktongue." *Journal of Nutrition* 14 (Oct. 1937) : 373–81.

———— and Julian M. Ruffin. "Pellagra Successfully Treated with Nicotinic Acid," *Journal of the American Medical Association* 109 (18 Dec. 1937), 2054–55.

———— and Julian M. Ruffin. "Pellagra Therapy." *New International Clinics* 2 (series 3, 1940), 103–14.

————. "Teaching Bacteriology as a Function of the Department of Medicine." *Southern Medical Journal* 27 (Aug. 1934) : 734–35.

————, Julian M. Ruffin, G. Margolis and L. H. Margolis. "Treatment of Experimental Canine Blacktongue and Clinical Pellagra with Coramine." *Journal of Clinical Investigation* 19 (Sept. 1940) : 775–76.

———— and Julian M. Ruffin. "The Use of Liver Extracts in the Treatment of Pellagra." *Transactions of the Medical Society of the State of North Carolina* 84 (1937) : 509–13.

Smith, Susan Gower. "A New Symptom Complex in Vitamin G Deficiency in Rats." *Proceedings of the Society for Experimental Biology and Medicine* 30 (Nov. 1932) : 198–200.

"Student Nurses Will Be College Girls at Duke University." *The Modern Hospital* 35 (Sept. 1930) : 105.

Taylor, Haywood M., and John S. Bradway. "The Teaching of Legal Medicine." *American Journal of Medical Jurisprudence* 2 (May-June 1939) : 210–13.

Voegtlin, Carl. "Recent Work on Pellagra." *Public Health Reports* 35 (18 June 1920) : 1435–52.

Walker, W. F. "What the Depression Has Done to Health Services." *Public Management* 16 (Nov. 1934) : 360–84.

Walters, W. "Discussion." *Annals of Surgery* 110 (Aug. 1939) : 308–09.

Wilbur, Ray L. "The Relationship of Medical Education to the Cost of Medical Care." *Journal of the American Medical Association* 92 (27 April 1929) : 1410–12.

Wyckoff, Ralph W. C. "Ultracentrifugal Concentration of a Homogenous Heavy Component from Tissues Diseased with Equine Encephalomyelitis." *Proceedings of the Society for Experimental Biology and Medicine* 36 (June 1937) : 771–73.

Zapffe, Fred C. "Analysis of Entrance Credentials of the Freshman Class, 1931–1932." *Journal of the Association of American Medical Colleges* 8 (Jan. 1933) : 40–45.

Books and Pamphlets

American Tobacco Company. *"Sold American"—The First Fifty Years*. New York: 1954.

Annual Report of the Trustees, Watts Hospital. 1895.

Ashe, Samuel A., ed. *Biographical History of North Carolina*. 8 vols. Greensboro, N.C.: Charles L. Van Noppen, 1905–1917.

Bachmeyer, Arthur C., ed. *The Hospital in Modern Society*. New York: The Commonwealth Fund, 1943.

Barber, Mary I., ed. *History of the American Dietetic Association*. Philadelphia: J. B. Lippincott Company, 1959.

Barrett, John G. *Sherman's March Through the Carolinas*. Chapel Hill: University of North Carolina Press, 1956.

Battle, Kemp B. *History of the University of North Carolina*. 3 vols. Raleigh: Edwards and Broughton, 1921.

Bernheim, Frederick. *The Interaction of Drugs and Cell Catalysts*. Minneapolis: Burgess Publishing Company, 1942.

Blackburn, William. *The Architecture of Duke University*. Durham: Duke University Press, 1939.

Boyd, William K. *The Story of Durham*. Durham: Duke University Press, 1927.

Bradway, John S. *Duke Legal Aid Clinic Annual Report*. 1 June 1939.

Burroughs, James A. *Needed Legislation and a Practical Enforcement of Existing Laws*. Asheville, N.C.: Furman & Messler, 1896.

Cameron, J. D. *A Sketch of the Tobacco Interests in North Carolina*. Oxford, N.C.: 1881.

Carson, Gerald. *The Roguish World of Dr. Brinkley*. New York: Holt, Rinehart and Winston, 1960.

Chaffin, Nora C. *Trinity College, 1839–1892: The Beginnings of Duke University*. Durham: Duke University Press, 1950.

Chamber of Commerce, Charlotte, N.C. *Charlotte as the Location of the Clinical Years of the Medical School of North Carolina*. Charlotte: 1922.

Clark, Paul. *James B. Duke and the Saugenay Region of Canada*. Privately printed, 1968.

Clark, Paul F. *The University of Wisconsin Medical School: A Chronicle, 1848–1948*. Madison: The University of Wisconsin Press, 1967.

The Commission on Graduate Medical Education. *Graduate Medical Education*. Chicago: University of Chicago Press, 1940.

The Commission on Medical Education. *Final Report of the Commission on Medical Education*. New York: Office of the Director of Study, 1932.

Corner, George W. *A History of the Rockefeller Institute*. New York: The Rockefeller Institute Press, 1964.

Crawford, Eugene B. *A History of Hospital Saving Association of North Carolina, Inc*. Chapel Hill: 1968.

Crowell, John Franklin. *A Program of Progress: An Open Letter to the General Assembly of North Carolina of 1891.* Trinity College: 1891.

———. *Personal Recollections of Trinity College, North Carolina: 1887–1894.* Durham: Duke University Press, 1939.

Cushing, Harvey. *The Life of Sir William Osler.* 2 vols. Oxford: The Clarendon Press, 1925.

Davis, Michael M. *Hospital Administration: A Career.* New York: The Rockefeller Foundation, 1929.

Davison, Wilburt C. *The Compleat Pediatrician.* Durham, 1934.

———. *The Duke University Medical Center, 1892–1960.* Durham: 1967.

———. *The First Twenty Years.* Durham: *Bulletin of Duke University* 24, no. 7–A: 1952.

Deitrich, John E., and Robert C. Berson. *Medical Schools in the United States at Mid-Century.* Evanston, Ill.: Association of American Medical Colleges, 1960.

Dickinson, Frank G., and James Ramond. *The Economic Position of Medical Care, 1929–1953.* Chicago: American Medical Association, 1955.

Durham Directory, 1907–1908. Durham: Hill Directory Company, 1907.

Durham, North Carolina, Chamber of Commerce. *Durham, North Carolina,* 1905.

Dwyer, M. Virginia, ed. *American Medical Directory, 1958.* Chicago: American Medical Association, 1958.

Falk, I. S., C. Rufus Rorem and M. D. Ring. *The Costs of Medical Care.* Publication no. 27 of The Committee on the Cost of Medical Care. Chicago: The University of Chicago Press, 1933.

Federal Support of Basic Research in Institutions of Higher Learning. Washington: National Academy of Sciences–National Research Council, 1964.

Few, William P. *The Duke Endowment and Duke University.* Durham, N.C.: Duke University, ca. 1930.

The First Two Years' Work of the Committee on the Cost of Medical Care. Washington: 1929.

The Five Year Program of the Committee on the Cost of Medical Care. Publication no. 1 of the Committee on the Cost of Medical Care. Washington: 1928.

Flexner, Abraham. *I Remember.* New York: Simon and Schuster, 1940.

———. "Medical Education in the United States and Canada," *Carnegie Foundation for the Advancement of Teaching Bulletin,* no. 4. Boston: The Mercymount Press, 1910.

Fosdick, Raymond B., with Henry F. Pringle and Katharine D. Pringle. *Adventure in Giving: The Story of the General Education Board.* New York: Harper and Row, 1962.

French, John C. *A History of the University Founded by Johns Hopkins.* Baltimore: The Johns Hopkins Press, 1946.

Garber, Paul N. *John Carlisle Kilgo.* Durham: Duke University Press, 1937.

Gelenas, Agnes. *Nursing and Nursing Education.* New York: The Commonwealth Fund, 1946.

Grisette, Felix A. *The Second Year: Annual Report of the Executive Director of Hospital Saving Association for the Year 1937.* Chapel Hill: 1938.

Hamblen, Edward C. *Endocrine Gynecology.* Springfield, Ill.: Charles C Thomas, 1939.

———. *Facts for Childless Couples.* Springfield, Ill.: Charles C Thomas, 1942.

Harris, Seale. *Clinical Pellagra.* St. Louis: The C. V. Mosby Company, 1941.

Indenture of James B. Duke Establishing the Duke Endowment, with Provisions of the Will and a Trust of Mr. Duke Supplementing the Same. Also an Address by William R. Perkins, Personal Counsel of Mr. Duke, on the Origin, Nature, and Purpose of the Duke Endowment. Charlotte: The Duke Endowment, 1932.

Interdepartment Committee to Coordinate Health and Welfare Activities. *The Nation's Health.* Washington: U.S. Government Printing Office, 1938.

Interdepartmental Committee to Coordinate Health and Welfare Activities. *A National Health Program: Report of the Technical Committee on Medical Care, 1938.* Washington: U.S. Government Printing Office, 1939.

Jenkins, John W. *James B. Duke, Master Builder.* New York: George H. Doran Company, 1927.

Johnston, Joseph E. *Narration of Military Operations.* Bloomington: University of Indiana Press, 1959.

Kilgo, John Carlisle. *The Lines of the Future Development of Trinity College.* 1902.

Lacy, B. R., Jr. *George W. Watts: The Seminary's Great Benefactor.* Durham: 1922.

Lefler, Hugh T. *History of North Carolina.* 2 vols. New York: Lewis Historical Publishing Company Inc., 1956.

Leland, R. G. *Distribution of Physicians in the United States.* Chicago: American Medical Association, 1935.

Lilly Research Laboratories: Dedication. Indianapolis, Indiana: Eli Lilly and Company, 1934.

Mayers, Lewis, and Leonard V. Harrison. *The Distribution of Physicians in the United States.* New York: General Education Board, 1924.

Medical Care for the American People. Publication no. 28 of The Committee on the Cost of Medical Care. Chicago: The University of Chicago Press, 1932.

Merton, Robert K., George G. Reader and Patricia L. Kendall, eds. *The Student Physician.* Cambridge: Harvard University Press, 1957.

Moulton, F. R., ed. *Aerobiology.* Washington: American Association for the Advancement of Science, 1942.

Munger, Claude W. *Report of a Study of the Lincoln Hospital.* Durham: 1947.

Myrdal, Gunnar. *An American Dilemma.* New York: Harper & Row, Publishers, 1962.

Paschal, George Washington. *History of Wake Forest College.* 3 vols. Wake Forest, N.C.: Wake Forest College, 1943.

Paul, Hiram V. *History of the Town of Durham, N.C.* Raleigh: Edwards and Broughton, 1884.

Pepper, George W. *Personal Recollections of Sherman's Campaigns in Georgia and the Carolinas.* Zanesville, Ohio: Hugh Dunne, 1866.

Perkins, William R. *An Address on the Duke Endowment: Its Origin, Nature and Purposes.* Charlotte: The Duke Endowment, 1929.

Poe, Clarence, ed. *Hospital and Medical Care for All Our People.* Raleigh: North Carolina Hospital and Medical Care Commission, 1947.

Porter, Earl W. *Trinity and Duke: 1892–1924.* Durham: Duke University Press, 1964.

Reed, Louis S. *The Ability to Pay for Medical Care.* Chicago: University of Chicago Press, 1933.

————. *Blue Cross and Medical Service Plans.* Washington: U.S. Public Health Service, 1947.

Report of the Committee on the School of Medicine and Hospital to the Board of Trustees of Duke University. 5 June 1937.

Rivers, Thomas M., et al. *Virus Diseases.* Ithaca, New York: Cornell University Press, 1943.

Robert, Joseph C. *The Story of Tobacco in America.* New York: Alfred A. Knopf, 1949.

————. *The Tobacco Kingdom.* Durham: Duke University Press, 1938.

The Rockefeller Foundation Annual Report for 1940. New York: 1940.

Rorem, C. Rufus. *Hospital Care Insurance.* Chicago: American Hospital Association, 1937.

Rosenman, Samuel I., ed. *The Public Papers and Addresses of Franklin D. Roosevelt.* 13 vols. New York: Random House, 1938–1950.

Ruffin, Julian M., et al. *Selected Papers.* 2 vols. Ephrate, Penn.: The Science Press, 1968.

Sherman, William T. *Memoirs of General William T. Sherman.* 2 vols. New York: D. Appleton & Co., 1931.

Shryock, Richard H. *The Development of Modern Medicine.* Philadelphia: University of Pennsylvania Press, 1936.

————. *The History of Nursing.* Philadelphia: W. B. Saunders Company, 1959.

————. *The Unique Influence of The Johns Hopkins University on American Medicine.* New York: Hafner Publishing Company, 1953.

Strong, Charles M. *History of Mecklenburg County Medicine.* Charlotte: News Printing House, 1929.

A Study of Mental Health in North Carolina. Ann Arbor, Michigan: 1937.

Terris, Milton, ed. *Goldberger on Pellagra.* Baton Rouge: Louisiana State University Press, 1964.

Tilley, Nannie May. *The Bright-Tobacco Industry.* Chapel Hill: University of North Carolina Press, 1948.

Van Noppen, Charles L., ed. *In Memoriam: George Washington Watts.* Greensboro, N.C.: DeVinne Press, 1922.

Way, J. H., and L. B. McBrayer. *Medical Colleges in North Carolina.* Pinehurst, N.C.: 1928.

Weiskotten, Herman G., et al. *Medical Education in the United States, 1934–1939.* Chicago: American Medical Association, 1940.

Williams, Pierce. *The Purchase of Medical Care Through Fixed Periodic Payment.* New York: National Bureau of Economic Research, 1932.

Wilson, Louis R. *The University of North Carolina, 1900–1930.* Chapel Hill: University of North Carolina Press, 1957.

Winkler, John K. *Tobacco Tycoon.* New York: Random House, 1942.

Woody, Robert H., ed. *The Papers and Addresses of William Preston Few.* With a biographical appreciation by Robert H. Woody. Durham: Duke University Press, 1951.

Young, James Harvey. *The Medical Messiahs.* Princeton, N.J.: Princeton University Press, 1967.

Young, William W. *The Story of the Cigarette.* New York: D. Appleton & Co., 1916.

Interviews[1]

Altvater, F. Vernon. 21 December 1968.
Beard, Joseph W., M.D. 25 February 1969.
Bernheim, Frederick, M.D. 26 February 1969, 21 May 1969.
Bernheim, Mary L. C., M.D. 26 February 1969, 21 May 1969.
Callaway, J. Lamar, M.D. 4 June 1969.
Carter, F. Bayard, M.D. 15 May 1969.
Cocke, Norman A., by Frank Rounds. 20 April 1963.
Davison, Wilburt C., M.D., by Frank Rounds. April 1964, May 1964.
Eadie, George S., M.D. 20 June 1969.
Forbus, Wiley D., M.D. 2 June 1965 (Department of Audio-Visual Education),
    8 April 1969, 16 May 1969.
Hart, Julian Deryl, M.D. 6 December 1968, 26 February 1969, 14 May 1969.
Heatherington, Duncan C., M.D. 26 May 1969.
Hill, George W. 7 April 1967, 20 November 1968.
Laprade, W. T. 20 April 1967.
Lee, A. C., by Frank Rounds. April 1963.
McBryde, Angus, M.D. 23 June 1969.
Persons, Elbert L., M.D. 22 May 1969.
Rankin, Watson S., M.D., by Frank Rounds, 11 January 1965.
Reeves, Robert J., M.D. 7 March 1967 (Department of Audio-Visual Educa-
    tion).
Ross, Robert A., M.D. 12 March 1969.
Ruffin, Julian M., M.D. 15 January 1969, 20 May 1969.
Smith, David T., M.D. 17 September 1965 (Department of Audio-Visual Educa-
    tion), 10 January 1969, 14 February 1969, 14 April 1969, 15 May 1969.
Wells, Warner L., M.D. 19 June 1969.

1. Typescripts of the interviews noted as by Frank Rounds are included in the
Duke Endowment Collection. Videotapes of those marked "Department of
Audio-Visual Education" are housed in that department of the Duke University
Medical Center.

Manuscripts[2]

John Franklin Crowell Papers
Wilburt C. Davison Collection (Duke University Medical Center Library)
Wilburt C. Davison Papers
Department of Plant Engineering and Maintenance Papers
Benjamin Newton Duke Papers
Duke Endowment Collection
Duke Endowment Papers (The Duke Endowment, Charlotte, North Carolina)
James B. Duke Papers
Duke University Archives
Duke University Department of Dietetics Papers (Duke University Medical
    Center)

Duke University Department of Hospital Administration Papers (Duke University Medical Center)

Duke University Medical Technology School Papers (Veterans Administration Hospital, Durham, North Carolina)

Duke University School of Nursing Papers (Duke University School of Nursing)

William Preston Few Papers

Robert L. Flowers Papers

Wiley D. Forbus Papers (In possession of Dr. Wiley D. Forbus, Durham, North Carolina)

Clarence E. Gardner, Jr., Papers

Oscar C. E. Hansen-Pruss Papers

John Sprunt Hill Papers (Papers in the possession of his son, George Watts Hill, Durham, North Carolina)

John Carlisle Kilgo Papers

Eugene Morehead Papers

North Carolina Blue Cross-Blue Shield Papers (North Carolina Blue Cross-Blue Shield, Inc., Durham, North Carolina)

Elbert L. Persons, Jr., Papers

Edward Featherston Small Papers

Trinity College Papers

Trustee Records, 1901–1922 (The classification includes memoranda, reports, treasurer's records, letters, working papers, and exhibits deposited in envelopes by years. Treasurer's Office of Duke University)

University Papers (Wilson Library: University of North Carolina at Chapel Hill)

Charles L. Van Noppen Papers

2. The collections are located in the Perkins Library of Duke University unless otherwise noted.

Minutes and Records

Duke University Hospital Accessions Book

Duke University Hospital Operation Books

Duke University Payroll Sheets

Minutes of the Board of Commissioners of the Town of Durham, North Carolina

Minutes of the Board of Trustees of Trinity College and Duke University, 1880–1933 (One volume, 1901–1910, was destroyed by fire in 1911. Offices of the Secretary and Treasurer of Duke University)

Minutes of the Board of Trustees of the University of North Carolina, with Minutes of the Executive Committee (Wilson Library: University of North Carolina)

Minutes of the Executive Committee of the Faculty of the Duke University School of Medicine

Minutes of the Meetings of the Board of Commissioners of Durham County, North Carolina

Minutes of the Meetings of the Board of Directors of the Hospital Care Associa-

tion, Incorporated (North Carolina Blue Cross-Blue Shield, Inc., Durham,
North Carolina)
Minutes of the Meetings of the Trustees of the Duke Endowment (The Duke
Endowment: Charlotte, North Carolina)
Minutes of the Trustees of Watts Hospital, 1895–1909 (Watts Hospital, Dur-
ham, North Carolina)

Newspapers

The Daily Tobacco Plant (Durham, North Carolina)
Durham Globe (Durham, North Carolina)
Durham Herald-Sun (Durham, North Carolina)
Durham Morning Herald (Durham, North Carolina)
Durham Recorder (Durham, North Carolina)
Durham Tobacco Plant (Durham, North Carolina)
Evening Sun (Baltimore, Maryland)
Greensboro Daily News (Greensboro, North Carolina)
Raleigh Christian Advocate (Raleigh, North Carolina)
Raleigh Morning Post (Raleigh, North Carolina)
Raleigh News and Observer (Raleigh, North Carolina)
State Chronicle (Raleigh, North Carolina)

Periodicals

Annual Register of Trinity College
Annual Report of the General Education Board
Bulletin of Duke University
Bulletin of the North Carolina Board of Health
The Duke Endowment: Annual Report of the Hospital Section. 1925–1939
The Duke Endowment: Yearbook. Nos. 1–4, 1924–1932
Transactions of the Medical Society of the State of North Carolina
Trinity Archive
University of North Carolina Record

Public Documents

North Carolina State Board of Health. *Biennial Report of the North Carolina
Board of Health to the General Assembly of North Carolina; Session 1877.*
Raleigh: P. M. Hale, 1877.
North Carolina State Board of Health. *Second Biennial Report of the North
Carolina Board of Health to the General Assembly of North Carolina; Ses-
sion 1889.* Raleigh: Edwards and Broughton, 1889.

U.S., Congress, House of Representatives. *Reports* no. 356. 69th Cong., 1st Sess., 1926.

U.S., Congress, Senate, Committee on Education and Labor. *Hearings, S. 3230.* 76th Cong., 3rd Sess., 1940.

U.S., Congress, Senate, Committee on Education and Labor. *Hearings, S. 191.* 79th Cong., 1st Sess., 1945.

U.S., *Statutes at Large.* vols. 43–44.

U.S. Bureau of the Census. *Fourteenth Census of the United States: 1920. Population,* vols. 1, 3, 4.

U.S. Bureau of the Census. *Thirteenth Census of the United States: 1910. Population,* vols. 3–4.

U.S. Bureau of Corporations. *Report of the Commissioner of Corporations on the Tobacco Industry.* 3 vols. Washington: U.S. Government Printing Office, 1909–15.

U.S. Census Office. *Twelfth Census of the United States: 1900. Population,* vol. 2.

U.S. Census Office. *Compendium of the Tenth Census 1880.* Washington: Government Printing Office, 1883.

U.S. Census Office. *Eleventh Census of the United States: 1890. Population,* vol. 2.

Theses and Dissertations

Cahow, Clark R. "The History of the North Carolina Mental Hospitals, 1848–1960." Ph.D. dissertation, Duke University, 1967.

Carpenter, Coy C. "A History of Wake Forest University in the Field of Medical Education with Personal Reminiscences by the Author." Unpublished material, 1968.

Griffin, Joseph E. "The Buzzard Roost Case." M.A. thesis, Duke University, 1941.

Herndon, Elisha M. "Early History of the Hospital Care Association, Incorporated." Unpublished paper in possession of author, 1968.

Index

Admissions: hospital, 83, 189; outpatient clinics, 83, 189; procedures, 71, 82, 91–93
Advertising: in medicine, 93–95; in tobacco industry, 4, 6, 7
Agricultural depression: and incidence of pellagra, 130; in 1890's, 16–19; in 1920's and 1930's, 79–80
Allen, George G., 41, 55, 72
Altvater, F. Vernon, 191; appointed Superintendent of Duke Hospital, 90; develops "flat rate" billing system, 90–93; with Hospital Care Association, 100–03
Aluminum Company of America, 35, 40 ff., 44, 55
Alyea, Edwin P., 64, 191
American blastomycosis: as subject of research, 134–38
American Civil War, 3–4
American College of Surgeons, 164, 167
American Dietetic Association, 160
American Hospital Association, 102
American Medical Association, 20, 29, 33, 68, 141
American Psychiatric Association, 177
American Tobacco Company: incorporated, 16; domination of tobacco industry, 16–17; dissolved by Supreme Court, 22–23
Amoss, Harold L., 45, 61–64, 69, 86, 159, 191
Anatomy, 13, 15, 48; as orienting students' attitudes toward medical studies, 109–10; as taught at Duke, 109–10
Anderson, William B., 191
Armstrong, W. H., 20
Arnett, Trevor, 65, 66

Bachmeyer, Arthur C., 173
Bacteriology: as taught at Duke, 111–12; blastomycosis, research in, 135–38
Baker, Bessie, 63, 64, 67, 69, 191
Baker, Roger D., 67, 191
Baptist Female Seminary (Meredith College), 12
Baptists, 19, 32, 183
Bassett, John S., 24
Batchelder, Marian F., 64
Beard, Dorothy, Research Fund, 153
Beard, Joseph W.: appointed, 151; research on equine encephalomyelitis, 151–54
Beds, 70, 190
Bell, William B., 151
Bennett, James, 3
Bernheim, Frederick, 154, 191; appointed, 67; research interests and methods, 149; teaching methods, 111; tuberculosis research, 150

Bernheim, Mary L. C., 149, 191
Biddle, Anthony, 41
Biochemistry: as taught at Duke, 110–11; student as subject in, 111
Biology, 16
Blackwell, William T., 4, 9; his tobacco company, 4
Blackwood, N. J., 166
Blue Cross plans, 99–103
Bonsack, James, 6–7, 9, 16
Botany, 13
Bowman Gray School of Medicine, 183
Bradford, William Z., 118
Brinkley, John R., 140, 141
Brooks, Eugene Clyde, 32
Bryson, E. W., 153
Bumpass, B. F., 13
Burkholder, C. F., 41
Butenandt, Adolph, 144, 154
Buttrick, Wallace, 24, 25, 28, 44

Callaway, J. Lamar, 115, 117
Canada, 35, 38, 39
Cansler, E. T., 41
Carey, D. T., 59
Carnegie, Andrew, 26
Carnegie Foundation, 25, 26
Carpenter, Coy C., 182
Carr, Albert G.: attempts to gain hospital and medical school for Durham, 8–14; role in founding of Lincoln Hospital, 20; role in founding of Watts Hospital, 19
Carr, Lewis A., 17
Carr, Julian S., 4, 10, 11, 13, 17
Carroll, Robert S., 177
Carter, Bayard, 154, 191; appointed, 67–68; research in vaginal flora, 138, 140; teaching methods, 118–19
Ceremonies, 75–76, 185
Chamber of Commerce, Charlotte, N.C., 30
Charity hospital care: and "flat rate" billing, 90–95; at Watts Hospital, 19, 95–96; cooperation with county governments, 95–98; in America, 79–81; need for at opening of Duke Hospital, 57–59; percentage of total care at Duke Hospital, 189; surveyed in Carolinas prior to founding of Duke Endowment, 37 ff.
Chase, H. W., 29, 30, 31, 32
Chemistry, 13, 15, 16
Christian, Henry A., 71
Clinical instruction: of interns, 119–22; of residents, 122–23; of undergraduates, 114–19